Natural PREGNANCY GUIDE

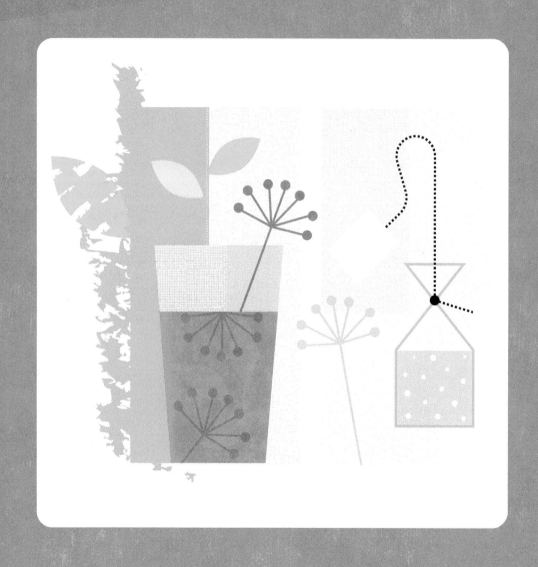

Natural
PREGNANCY
GUIDE

EMPOWERING MOMS TO MAKE HEALTHY CHOICES

LAURENA WHITE

MD, L.Ac.

Illustrations by Bee Murphy

ROCKRIDGE
PRESS

For general information on our other products and services or to obtain technical support, please contact our Customer Care Department within the United States at (866) 744-2665, or outside the United States at (510) 253-0500.

Rockridge Press publishes its books in a variety of electronic and print formats. Some content that appears in print may not be available in electronic books, and vice versa.

Interior and Cover Designer: Patricia Fabricant
Art Producer: Hannah Dickerson
Editor: Mo Mozuch
Production Editor: Ruth Sakata Corley
Illustrations © 2020 Bee Murphy. Photography © Darren Muir, p. 64; Tanya Zouev/StockFood, p. 87; Ina Peters/Stocksy, p. 106. Author photo courtesy of Robert Perilla.

ISBN: Print 978-1-64739-707-4 | eBook 978-1-64739-708-1
R0

I dedicate this book to all
the people in this world who
desire to experience the gift and
the process of becoming a mother.
My hope is that this book awakens
you to the beauty and all the
possibilities that lie ahead during
pregnancy, labor, and delivery.
May you discover the strength
that lies within you . . . right
there in your womb.

Contents

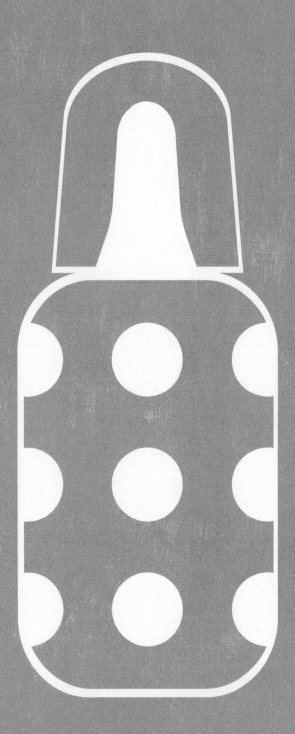

Introduction

Welcome! By opening this book, you are opening the door to new concepts while educating yourself on a variety of pregnancy-related topics. You will be surprised by how much you learn as you emerge empowered with knowledge.

Pregnancy is a physiological (normal, bodily) process. As an integrative health practitioner, I combine the essential aspects of Western (conventional) and Eastern (traditional) medicine in a reproductive medicine and women's health practice. In this way I can call on Mother Nature to support this often-medicalized period in a woman's life. Many women today opt for an intervention-free, nonmedicated pregnancy (and birth), much like popular diets today use *organic, clean, whole, and plant-based* eating to minimize toxins entering the body. In my practice, I work with mothers who want to give their babies the healthiest beginnings possible and make intentional efforts to avoid the toxins that can be found in food, hormones, and pharmaceutical drugs.

Although artificial fertility treatments can help you conceive, pregnancy itself is a spontaneous bodily process. Childbirth is the *natural* outcome of pregnancy, but the vague term "natural childbirth" shames women whose deliveries require medication or surgical intervention. By allowing labor to progress as it was designed to do, a woman can control, to some extent, the emotional and physical aspects of labor and her own memory of the birth experience. Weighing the risks and benefits, being honest about what makes you feel comfortable (and uncomfortable), and then moving forward with confidence is the tangible part of pregnancy that empowers you on the path to motherhood.

How to Use This Book

This book serves as a guide to help expectant mothers make decisions; however, it does not push any one point of view over another. A "one-size-fits-all" approach doesn't work here. Just as every person is an individual with specific needs, wants, and desires, each woman's pregnancy will be different from her previous pregnancies, and will definitely differ from anyone else's. The goal of this book is to guide women through their own unique pregnancy and childbirth experiences in the healthiest way possible.

Believe it or not, the current cost of health care means that an unmedicated pregnancy without medical interventions will actually be more expensive than a "traditional" pregnancy. Out-of-pocket consultations cost more than appointments directly covered by insurance. Parents who want an unmedicated pregnancy and birth should plan accordingly, using tax-advantaged Flexible Spending Accounts (FSA) or Health Savings Accounts (HSA) to cover appointments and related expenses. (The planning ahead doesn't end after the birth, either!) In much the same way, organic diet and lifestyle choices can always be substituted with less-expensive, nonorganic versions, but they don't offer the same "natural" benefits. Luckily, there are resources out there to help; the Environmental Working Group (EWG.org), for example, maintains "Clean Fifteen" and "Dirty Dozen" lists that highlight key foods that can be purchased in nonorganic form.

Part 1 covers the importance of establishing, maintaining, and practicing healthy habits throughout your pregnancy and beyond. Part 2 and part 3 offer specific guidance for managing symptoms and dealing with challenges you may encounter during your pregnancy journey. Make sure you keep your provider in the loop about any medical decisions in order to keep your safety and the safety of your newborn front and center.

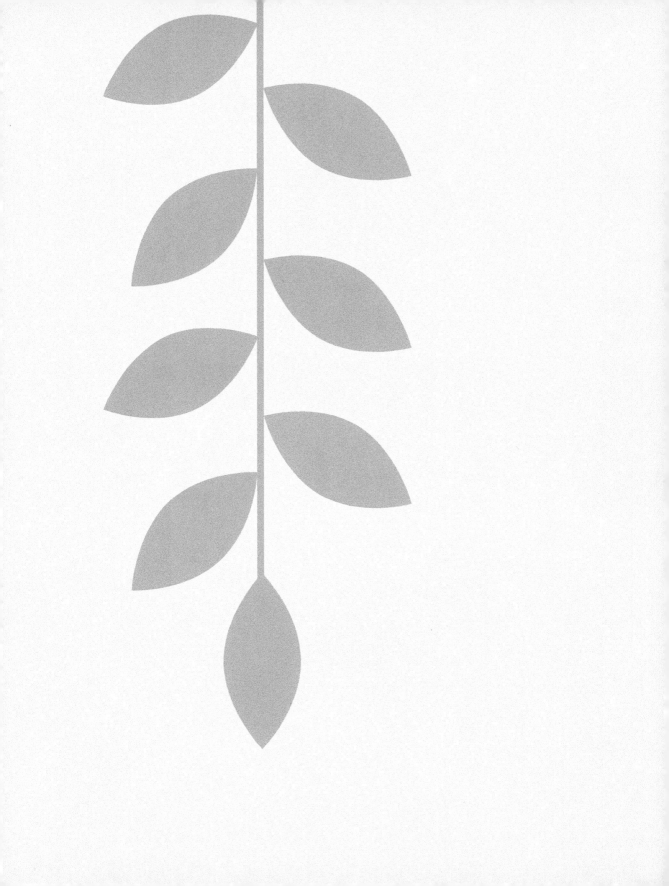

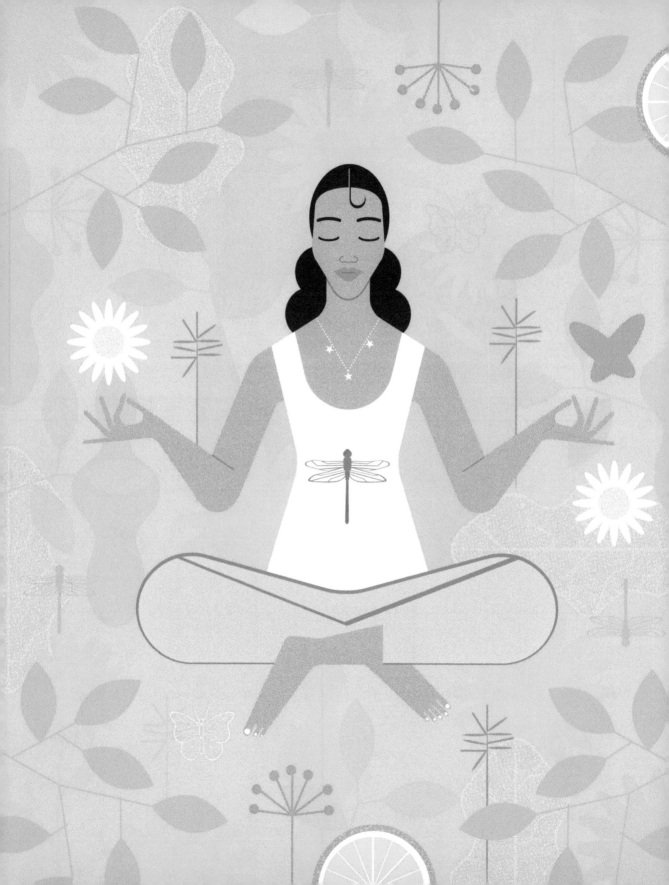

Part One

GETTING BACK TO NATURAL

You're pregnant! Congratulations!

Your pregnant body goes through a number of changes as it adapts to the needs of your growing baby. Many women choose pregnancy as the time to begin a detoxification process out of concern for their child's future health. Ironically, though, the best time for detoxification is six weeks to three months *prior* to pregnancy. Since a genuine detox process involves making strict dietary changes, it can actually stimulate toxins as they circulate through your bloodstream. Since your blood is what your body uses to feed your baby, these changes can have negative effects on your baby's development. Starting this intense process *before* conceiving allows a woman to focus on making healthy changes—particularly for liver and gut health—without harming her baby.

The following section offers information about *cleansing* your system in gentle ways during your pregnancy, making healthy choices in makeup selections, skin care regimens, and cleaning products, while avoiding and eliminating toxins and pesticides in your car, home, and work environments. It also includes tips on establishing new healthy habits during pregnancy, including improvements in diet and nutrition, relaxation techniques, and pregnancy-safe exercises.

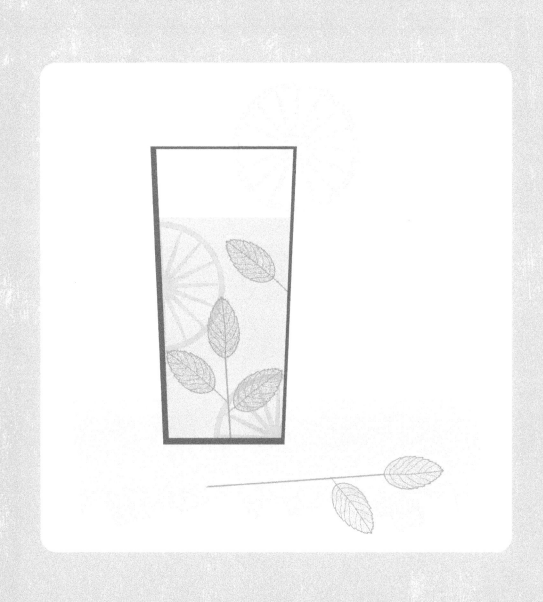

CHAPTER ONE

Detoxify Your Life

While undergoing a physical detox at the beginning of your pregnancy is not recommended, now is the ideal time to detoxify your home. This process may seem overwhelming as you learn about the toxins that can affect your baby in utero, but this book can help guide you. From skin care products and household cleaners to paint and mattresses, you'll become a pro at recognizing the different chemicals and products to avoid.

To limit your exposure and keep your growing family healthy, start in your bathroom. Now is the time to read labels and purge your home of toxic chemicals found in cosmetics, sunscreens, and household cleaners, replacing them with safer, green options. Protect your baby from household electromagnetic fields (EMF) by educating yourself on the types of EMFs. As you design the nursery, carefully choose the paint and the finish on your furniture, since volatile organic compounds (VOCs) can emit toxins from the crib, bed, mattresses, and rugs. Your goal now is to create a nurturing environment for your newborn, which will give you peace of mind, while you do your part to reduce the negative environmental effects of these toxins.

What We Mean by a Natural Pregnancy

Knowledge builds confidence, and being knowledgeable about your pregnancy is no exception. As pregnancy is already a natural process, it is important to work with it naturally. Being confident in your ability to have a safe and healthy pregnancy will help you successfully embark on your journey toward motherhood. A woman's body is designed for the experiences of pregnancy, labor, and childbirth. However, these experiences are less about enacting your birth plan and more about your overall approach, including eating healthy foods, drinking enough water, exercising properly, adapting to new postures, alleviating stress, and keeping yourself mentally healthy.

A healthy pregnancy includes creating a healthy environment, both in and out of the womb. Be intentional about setting aside time for yourself and your growing baby. Pay attention to how you are feeling emotionally, physically, and spiritually. Listen to yourself. Trust what your body is telling you. As you gather knowledge throughout your pregnancy, listen to the positive birth stories of other mothers you know and trust. Establishing your support system and determining your health care team is essential early on in pregnancy, as these people will offer you the love, wisdom, and inspiration you need along the way. Take the time to consider what ideal care looks like for you and your baby. Select a provider who makes you feel comfortable, knowing that this person will consciously, safely, and intentionally guide you through each step of your pregnancy with patience and confidence, just as nature intended.

The Birth Plan: Natural or No?

Your birth plan is your voice and it affects you and your baby. This is an opportunity to really think about what you want for yourself and for your newborn, both during childbirth and after delivery. Communicating your intentions to your team opens up the discussion and keeps all parties (providers, nurses, assistants, doulas, and family) in the loop. Now is the time to consider all your options. Taking the time to examine what's important to you and providing input regarding your care reflects your preferences. This is an empowering task, especially if you're aiming for a nonmedicated birth (if possible).

The popularity of nonmedicated birth stems from safety and health concerns for both mother and baby. Although pain is part of nonmedicated and medicated deliveries alike, nonmedicated childbirth gives the mother a heightened sense of clarity during the process, along with an easier and faster recovery. If you are considering a nonmedicated delivery, chapter 7 provides more information. No matter what your intentions are, every pregnant woman should think about a birth plan so that she can begin making the necessary arrangements. Unique medical situations, cost, location, and access to resources will all play a role. Keep in mind that you are no more of a mother if you choose to have a nonmedicated birth and no less of a mother if you choose painkillers or an epidural, or have a cesarean delivery.

Detox Safety

Pregnancy means dietary adjustments even for the healthiest woman. It can be tempting to try to cleanse your body after learning of your pregnancy, but popular cleanses (commercial and otherwise) can be aggressive and potentially harmful to you and your developing baby. Whereas strict diets are usually not necessary, mindful eating will become increasingly more important. Using the acronym SLOW (seasonal, local, organic, and whole) will help you stick to minimally processed foods while avoiding foods that are higher in additives, preservatives, pesticides, hormones, and other chemicals.

Before beginning any new regimen or detoxification program, talk to your health care provider. Multivitamins and supplements may or may not be necessary—and they are not all created equal. Avoid detox treatments that include fasting (intermittent or otherwise), dieting or calorie restriction, unpasteurized juices or milk, and specific time frames. While herbal therapy sounds healthier than synthetic drugs, it may not be. Whenever adding herbal remedies (including teas) to your nutrition regimen, please consult a licensed herbalist who is trained in herbal dosing as well as potentially harmful situations. Talk to your health care provider about herbal remedies, too.

There are gentle methods for clean eating during pregnancy. You can safely protect yourself and your baby from toxic, processed foods during pregnancy without using drastic detox methods. Avoiding synthetic products such as perfumes, fragrances, and plastics will also go a long way toward minimizing exposure to toxic chemicals without putting your baby through an intense detoxification process. Detox programs are unlikely to remove toxins any better than the body can do on its own anyway, and during pregnancy they can be potentially dangerous.

Water, Water Everywhere

Establishing healthy hydration habits early on in pregnancy is vital. Water helps pregnant women form amniotic fluid, the protective liquid contained by the amniotic sac. Amniotic fluid serves as a cushion for the growing fetus and facilitates the exchange of nutrients between mother and baby. In addition, water helps a pregnant woman produce extra blood, form new tissue, eliminate toxic waste (through urine, fecal matter, and sweat), and support digestive processes. Although drinking at least 80 ounces of water every day helps flush toxins out of the body, 112 ounces is ideal.

Keep in mind that all water is not created equal, even in the United States. Contact your local health department to find out where your drinking water comes from, especially if you drink water from a built-in refrigerator mechanism. Consider investing in a home water-purifying system if you don't have one, and, if it's an option, buy bottled water.

How will you know if you're hydrated enough? On your frequent trips to the restroom, look at the color of your urine. Pale yellow or clear urine means optimal hydration. Proper hydration helps decrease urinary tract infections, constipation, and hemorrhoids. More important, staying hydrated decreases your chances of preterm labor and preterm birth. If drinking enough water was challenging for you prior to pregnancy, infusing your water with frozen fruits such as lemons, raspberries, and limes could help. Try the following techniques if you want to avoid overheating, fatigue, and headaches.

LEMON WATER

Lemons are a wonderful source of magnesium, calcium, potassium, and vitamin C, important nutrients for a pregnant woman's bone health and a baby's brain development. Staying hydrated can get tedious, so keep things interesting by putting washed lemon wedges or lemon juice in your room temperature (or slightly warmer) water to boost its flavor. Slicing a lemon or scratching its peel may ward off the nausea associated with morning sickness. Adding Lemon essential oil to a diffuser can also be helpful. Keeping a vial of Lemon essential oil in your purse may be a viable alternative when you feel queasy throughout the day and you aren't at home. Merely inhaling the scent (directly from the vial or small bottle) will provide almost instant relief. However, be mindful of ingesting larger doses of Lemon essential oil (more than two drops per serving) since too much lemon can damage tooth enamel and trigger heartburn. Inhaling the scent is the preferable method as it more efficiently calms the symptoms of nausea. Moderation is key. As always, discuss your dietary concerns with your health care provider.

SPA WATER

Water is the ultimate purifier, hydrator, and replenisher. For expectant mothers, *spa water*, reminiscent of a relaxing spa day, is a popular choice. Basic spa water is made with lemon, cucumbers, and mint to create a gentle cleansing beverage. Be careful, though—mint has muscle relaxant properties, and if it's taken at the wrong time during pregnancy, it can relax the uterine muscles, inducing preterm labor or delivery. If you have had a previous miscarriage, it may be best to stay away from mint during your pregnancy.

Antioxidant-rich cucumbers cool inflammation in the body while promoting hydration, lowering blood sugar, and promoting gastrointestinal regularity. Water infused with fruits such as strawberries, watermelon, and blueberries, along with raw herbs like basil, can provide increased nutritional benefits through naturally added vitamins and minerals. Overnight infusion guarantees a delicious flavor.

RED RASPBERRY LEAF TEA

Red raspberry leaf, the "woman's herb," is especially beneficial for pregnant women. Although some pregnant women use this herbal remedy in the first trimester, the best time to start drinking the tea is at 32 weeks, giving it enough time to build to healthy levels in the body without any ill effects. One to three cups a day of tea in the third trimester can lead to a shorter first stage (thinning and opening of the cervix) or shorter second stage of labor (when the baby moves through the birth canal). Fragarine, the compound found in red raspberry leaves, helps tone the womb. The American Pregnancy Association also states that drinking the tea helps make delivery easier, reduces interventions, improves labor outcomes, decreases instrumentation, and prevents excessive postpartum bleeding. Consult your provider before using this tea during pregnancy. Discontinue drinking if you begin to spot or if Braxton Hicks contractions occur before the third trimester.

Supplement Your Water

Adding supplements to your water can help increase its cleansing potential. For example, if you're already beginning your day with lemon water, adding grated ginger can enhance the gentle cleansing properties of this drink. The lemon water and ginger work together to improve digestion and metabolism, and make an effective gentle cleanse when taken on an empty stomach. In this section, you'll read about key supplements that aid in the gentle cleansing process and are safe for women to take during the early stages of pregnancy. As always, talk to your provider about dosage before incorporating into your diet.

- DANDELION (*Taraxacum officinale*). Dandelion leaves can be used in formulas to stimulate appetite during pregnancy and to promote lactation in preparation for breastfeeding immediately after delivery. It also helps with fluid retention. Avoid dandelion leaves if taking lithium, diuretics, or antidiabetic medication.

- FLAX (*Linum usitatissimum*). Fiber-rich flaxseed is a natural laxative, relieving pregnancy constipation and hemorrhoids. It also helps control blood sugar levels, which often rise during pregnancy. Taking two tablespoons of ground flaxseed with food can reduce the likelihood of gestational diabetes, meaning your baby is less likely to have a high birth weight and resulting cesarean delivery.

- MILK THISTLE (*Silybum marianum*). Milk thistle protects and supports the liver in clearing excess hormones and toxins. A liquid extract preparation containing 70 to 80 percent silymarin helps prevent morning sickness. Drinking one to three cups of tea daily will also provide relief. Just simmer one teaspoon of milk thistle seeds in one cup of water for 10 minutes.

Break Up with Makeup

You may already be displaying clearer skin, compliments of your natural "pregnancy glow." Many women become more vigilant about what they are putting in their bodies once they become pregnant, but they may be less likely to think about what they are putting *on* their bodies. Adapting skin care regimens and using healthier cosmetic products help eliminate the readily absorbed toxins that are placed on your body, and also help accommodate the hormonal changes evident in your hair, skin, and nails. During pregnancy and while breastfeeding, avoid products containing the following chemicals:

BISPHENOL A'S (BPA) intensely toxic effects harm developing fetuses and babies more than any other age group. BPA contaminates liquid baby formula sold in metal cans. Over the first six months, milk comprises the entirety of your baby's diet. By choosing BPA-free formula and breastfeeding, you eliminate this exposure.

BUTYLATED HYDROXYANISOLE/HYDROXYTOLUENE (BHA/BHT) are preservatives generally recognized as safe by the FDA. However, several other state, national, and federal agencies have classified them both as endocrine disruptors and known carcinogens (cancer-causing substances) based on animal studies. Avoid chips, preserved meats, and flavorings that contain BHT, particularly those that also contain BHA.

COAL TAR DYES are a known cancer-causing agent found in shampoo and permanent hair dyes. These dyes last in the hair until the hair is cut off and have been linked to birth defects. In the United States, unfortunately, coal tar dyes do not need FDA approval.

DEA (DIETHANOLAMINE)-RELATED INGREDIENTS are derived from the DEA compound; however, they are not chemically the same as DEA. With that caveat, shampoos, soaps, and body products that contain DEA-derivatives have been prohibited in California. Avoid oleamide DEA, lauramide DEA, and cocamide DEA, cancer-causing agents especially harmful to pregnant women.

DIETHYL PHTHALATE (DEP) ranks among a group of undisclosed ingredients that have hazardous properties. Using certain cosmetics such as popular perfumes, colognes, and body sprays may expose you and your fetus to DEP, which can cause abnormal development of male reproductive organs, including permanent sperm damage.

FORMALDEHYDE-RELEASING PRESERVATIVES are known cancer-causing agents that increase your chances of having a miscarriage, so intentionally reducing exposure is an integral part of a healthy pregnancy. These preservatives can be found in blush, mascara, lotion, shampoo, sunscreen, moisturizer, conditioner, eyeshadow, nail polish, nail treatments, body wash, and makeup remover.

FRAGRANCES pass directly from the skin to the bloodstream. Hand lotions and lip gloss include synthetic fragrances that are highly toxic. They also include cancer-causing ingredients that are linked with reproductive birth defects. In cosmetic products, interpret the words "fragrance" and "parfum" as "hidden chemicals" and opt for fragrance-free products.

PARABENS (methylparaben, propylparaben, butylparaben, and ethylparaben), chemicals used as artificial preservatives in makeup, moisturizers, hair care products, and shaving products, disrupt hormones, harm fertility, affect birth outcomes, and increase the risk of cancer. Since quality products can be made safely without parabens, avoiding cosmetic products that contain them is paramount.

PETROLATUM is the main ingredient in most of the beauty products women use. Whereas properly refined petrolatum is not harmful, petrolatum is not fully refined in the United States and it contains toxic cancer-causing chemicals. To avoid products with petrolatum, only use products that contain fully refined white petrolatum.

PHTHALATES are found in nail polish, hair spray, and perfume. When these compounds pass to the fetus, abnormal sexual development can result. Fetuses exposed to phthalates are more likely to be born with hypospadias, a congenital condition where the opening of the penis is on the underside, or experience premature breast development later in life.

POLYETHYLENE GLYCOL (PEG) COMPOUNDS can be found in every class of personal care product, including but not limited to shampoo, sunscreen, face and body lotions, and makeup. Although these compounds range from nontoxic to highly toxic, some specific products release carcinogens while others can cause birth defects.

RETINOIDS have been linked to development and reproductive toxicity, ranging from infertility and reproductive organ cancers to birth defects and developmental delays in children. Products that include retinoids are SPF-containing moisturizers, serums, eye creams, antiaging products, body-firming lotions, bronzers, foundation, sunscreens, hairstyling aids, body washes, facial masks, cleansers, and depilatories.

SILOXANES are found most often in hair products, deodorants, sunscreens, moisturizers, and facial treatments. They are considered hormone disruptors that are toxic to the reproductive system and can cause uterine tumors. To avoid siloxanes, stay away from products that list "methicone" on the label.

SODIUM LAURETH SULFATE (not to be confused with Sodium *lauryl* sulfate) is salient in a large swath of cosmetic and beauty products, including hand soap, shampoo, body wash, and toothpaste. Not only is this compound carcinogenic, but it can also cause birth defects. Look for sodium laureth sulfate–free products.

TRICLOSAN, commonly found in toothpaste and facial cleansers, is merely accompanied by use recommendations and manufacturing restrictions in the United States. In other countries, triclosan is prohibited (Canada) or accompanied by specific concentration restrictions (Japan). Multiple studies have shown that triclosan is a hormone disruptor in low doses.

How to Stay Clean and Green

Maintaining a clean home during pregnancy is challenging, but it can also be downright dreadful, especially when using harsh cleaning products. Noxious fumes can be triggering for your heightened sense of smell, and the harsh chemical odors can exacerbate morning sickness. In addition, prenatal exposure to aerosol and spray bottle cleaners are associated with an increased risk of childhood asthma. If inhaled or swallowed, certain chemicals can enter the bloodstream and pass to your baby through the placenta. Your baby can also be exposed to chemicals after birth through your breast milk.

Many commercial brands of cleaning agents (even the "green" ones) contain chemical ingredients that should be avoided during the first trimester of pregnancy, which is an important period of fetal brain and spinal cord development.

As hormone disruptors, these chemicals can increase the risk of pregnancy complications, congenital abnormalities, birth defects, and even cancer. Surprisingly and unfortunately, the toxic chemicals are usually not printed on the product labels. Although eliminating exposure to all harmful environmental toxins when you're pregnant would be impossible, you can reduce regular exposure to these chemicals with the following homemade cleaning products:

- **ALL-PURPOSE CLEANER.** Adding 20 drops of Citrus essential oil to ½ cup of white vinegar and 2 cups of water creates an antibacterial and germicidal cleaner.

- **MOLD AND MILDEW CLEANER.** If possible, avoid cleaning mold and mildew altogether when pregnant. To clean it naturally, use white distilled vinegar to penetrate porous materials. Spray on a surface, let it sit for a few minutes, rinse, and dry.

- **WINDOW CLEANER.** Combine 2 cups of water, ¼ cup of white vinegar, and ¼ teaspoon of dishwashing liquid in a spray bottle. Use newspaper to eliminate streaks.

- **WOOD CLEANER.** Mix ½ cup of white vinegar, ¼ cup of olive oil, 1 tablespoon each of lemon juice and vegetable glycerin, and 25 drops of essential oil.

Dry Brushing

Skin is the largest organ in our body. During pregnancy, your skin deserves an energy boost. Dry brushing is a self-care practice that involves brushing your skin with a dry, firm, plant-based, bristled brush with long, slow strokes before bathing. After brushing your entire body, take a shower or bath and pat your body dry. Then you can massage your favorite organic oil onto your skin, leaving your body feeling completely revitalized.

Dry brushing feels great, smooths and exfoliates skin, cleans and reduces pores, helps minimize cellulite, prevents stretch marks, and stimulates blood flow, all while supporting your lymphatic system, which helps rid the body of waste. As circulation improves, your skin becomes softer and your immune system gets stronger. As with any new regimen during pregnancy,

AVOID THE LITTER BOX

Toxoplasmosis is an infection caused by a parasite that can live in undercooked, contaminated meat or shellfish. It's also found in water and soil that has been contaminated with cat feces that contains the *Toxoplasma gondii* parasite, so wear gloves when gardening and wash your hands with soap and water afterward.

Toxoplasmosis transmitted through cat feces may lead to miscarriage. As such, the cat litter box should be changed daily. Expectant mothers should try to avoid changing the cat litter box, but if you have to do it, wear disposable gloves and wash your hands right away with soap and water. While you're pregnant, keep your cat indoors, only feed your cat dry or canned food, and do not adopt a new cat or kitten (outdoor or stray), as they are more likely to have eaten raw meat.

If you become infected with toxoplasmosis during (or just before) your pregnancy, you can pass the infection to your baby even if you are asymptomatic. Although infected infants do not usually have symptoms at birth, blindness or mental disabilities may develop during childhood.

If a nursing mother has mastitis and cracked or bleeding nipples soon after an infection when the parasite is still in her bloodstream, she *could* transmit the infection to her baby; however, transmitting the infection through breast milk is unlikely.

talk to your provider before starting this self-care routine. Be extra gentle during pregnancy, especially around your lower abdomen and stomach. Make sure that your long, slow strokes are very light, or you can avoid this region altogether if it's not comfortable, focusing on your feet, legs, hands, arms, buttocks, hips, and back. During the postpartum period (the "fourth trimester"), dry brushing can also help reduce the appearance of both new and old stretch marks by tightening your postpartum skin and increasing the absorption of creams and lotions. So even if your provider suggests that you postpone dry brushing until after your baby is born, you can still create a daily postpartum self-care ritual by incorporating this all-natural practice.

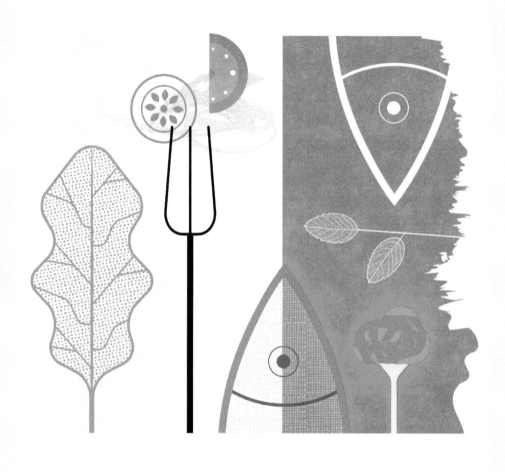

CHAPTER TWO

Nutrition and Diet

The statement, attributed to Hippocrates, "Let thy food be thy medicine and thy medicine be thy food," is the most important lifestyle intervention that you can adopt at this point in your pregnancy. Along with regularly scheduled prenatal care, eating foods that are not only healthy but specifically healthy for *you* is a prerequisite for the health and wellness of your baby. Women who exercise regularly and eat a diet that is appropriate for their blood type and body type are less likely to experience pregnancy complications and are more likely to give birth to a healthy baby. A well-balanced diet reduces the risks of unwanted pregnancy symptoms such as anemia, mood swings, morning sickness, and fatigue.

Even though the majority of your nutrients will come from solid food during pregnancy, a quality prenatal vitamin will provide a boost to an already nutritious diet. Prenatal vitamins serve a specific purpose and do not replace daily nutrient-rich meals.

Having aversions to certain foods while craving other foods (sweets, fast food, carbohydrates, and fatty foods) are common occurrences during pregnancy. Even though this is a popularly held belief, food cravings are *not* your body's way of telling you what it needs. Giving in to cravings may actually be harmful to you and your fetus because of the unnecessary weight gain. Mindfulness and intentionally refocusing help women make more wholesome food selections. This chapter provides insight into the best foods to eat, the necessary supplements to take (and avoid), and where the risks lie in term of pesticides and genetically modified organisms.

Eating According to Your Blood Type

Eating right for your blood type is a concept created by naturopath Peter J. D'Adamo, which supports eating foods that react chemically with your blood type in positive ways. Unlike most restriction diets, which eliminate large swaths of entire food groups from every person's diet, here food is broken down into twelve food groups (beans/legumes, beverages/tea/coffee, condiments/sweeteners/additives, dairy/eggs, fruit, grains/cereals, herbs/spices, meats/poultry, nuts/seeds, oils/fats, seafood, and vegetables) and then further separated into *beneficial, neutral,* and *avoid* categories.

- People with TYPE O blood are guided toward a diet high in protein, heavy on lean meat, poultry, fish, and vegetables, and light on grains, beans, and dairy, since the last triggers digestive issues, weight gain, and other health concerns.

- Those with TYPE A blood are on the opposite end of the spectrum and should eat a meat-free diet based on fruits and vegetables, beans and legumes, and whole grains (organic and fresh) due to their sensitive immune systems.

- If you have TYPE B blood, avoiding corn, wheat, buckwheat, lentils, tomatoes, peanuts, sesame seeds, and chicken will help you maintain a healthy weight, while eating green vegetables, eggs, certain meats, and low-fat dairy will boost your overall health and wellness.

Lastly, those with TYPE AB blood should incorporate tofu, seafood, dairy, and green vegetables into their diets. Since they tend to have low stomach acid, they should also avoid caffeine, alcohol, and smoked or cured meats.

Keep in mind that these recommendations can be modified easily, with substitutions that will stretch your palate in different ways if you are willing to make the effort. Initially, eating according to blood type seems "restrictive" and can be challenging for some people, given that some entire food groups are not *beneficial* for some blood types (e.g., meat is not *beneficial* for those with type A blood); however, there are *neutral* options available. Similarly, there are foods in the *avoid* category in each group that might not cause you any *apparent* problems when eaten in moderation.

Adopting this way of eating is definitely a lifestyle change, not just a fad diet. It can be modified based on your personal tastes and specific health challenges. However, our practice has found that many sensitivities (gluten and dairy specifically) align with blood type, and eating accordingly helps minimize symptoms of chronic conditions like diabetes, high cholesterol, and high blood pressure without using costly supplements and lifelong medication.

Although there is historical context for each blood type in terms of food, there are other aspects of the eating-right-for-your-type lifestyle that include stress management, exercises, and lifestyle strategies, which help integrate the mind, body, and spirit . . . central tenets of healing.

The Superfoods

Nutrient-dense foods are the most favorable sources of baby-building nourishment. Even though you are not actually "eating for two," you will routinely need additional calories, especially in the second trimester. Since all foods are not created equal, the foods you put in your body to benefit you and your unborn child will be the most important daily decisions you make. Eating for your blood type, for example, ensures maximum benefits for you and your baby. Some expectant mothers will also need to follow specific diets designed to help pregnancy-induced conditions like gestational diabetes and intrauterine growth restriction. These diets in particular help women keep their blood sugar levels within the normal range and consume a healthy number of daily calories. For your overall health and well-being as well as that of your developing baby, here are some common "superfoods" to consider adding to your diet.

BERRIES are filled with vitamin C, which improves iron absorption, potassium, folate, and, most important, antioxidants, which protect against cellular damage. Raspberries are high in fiber while cranberries help prevent urinary tract infections. Despite these amazing benefits, many women do not meet the pregnancy fruit requirements. Adding just one to two cups of berries per day to your diet will help prevent miscarriage and preeclampsia by combating inflammation. Whether on top of cereal, layered with yogurt parfait-style, in smoothies, on salads, or alone, eating berries after a high-protein meal helps you absorb nutrients and enhances the brain health of your child.

DARK GREEN LEAFY VEGETABLES AND BROCCOLI are unique superfoods in that they contain most of the nutrients pregnant women need. They are rich in fiber, which helps prevent and resolve constipation, and also high in other nutrients like folate, calcium, lutein, potassium, vitamin A, and carotenoids. You can easily incorporate dark, leafy green vegetables and broccoli into pasta, soups and stews, and stir-fry dishes. They can also simply be roasted or sautéed for added flavor.

DATES are the quintessential nutritious and healthy pregnancy snack. They are a source of iron, vitamin K, potassium, and folate, which helps reduce birth defects. As dates are naturally sweet, they offer a healthier alternative to satisfying your sweet tooth than other craving options. Additionally, dates are fiber-rich, which helps prevent pregnancy-related constipation. Eating dates also enhances the labor experience. Six dates a day during the last four weeks of pregnancy ripens the cervix prior to delivery. Depending on how many dates you eat, labor could start without the help of medication, since dates are believed to induce labor naturally.

DIGESTIVE AIDS that address constipation can also come in beverage form. Like water, 100 percent fruit juice softens stools and keeps the bowels moving. As prunes are a known natural laxative, a cup of prune juice each morning will help maintain regularity. For a gentler laxative effect, try apple juice. Pear juice is another great option; it is not as rich in vitamins as prune juice, but it contains four times more sorbitol, a natural laxative, than apple juice does. Many women prefer apple and pear flavors over the flavor of prune juice.

ENZYME-RICH FOODS aid the digestive process by breaking down fats, proteins, and carbohydrates into easily absorbed molecules. Pineapples contain bromelain; ripe, raw papayas contain papain; ginger contains zingibain; and kiwifruit contains actinidain, all of which help break down proteins. Kiwifruit eases bloating and constipation while ginger helps food move faster through the digestive tract. Mangos, bananas, and raw honey contain amylase, which breaks down carbohydrates. Avocados and kefir, a fermented milk, contain lipase, which breaks down fat while populating your body with beneficial bacteria. Sauerkraut (fermented cabbage), kimchi (fermented vegetables), and miso (fermented soybeans) have probiotic properties that ease digestive symptoms.

LEGUMES are an economical source of protein, fiber, and folate. Folate is a critical nutrient during pregnancy and reduces the risk of neural tube and birth defects. Chickpeas are great for homemade hummus. Black beans are usually associated with rice and soups and are high in antioxidants, fiber, and magnesium. Lentils come in several colors, and one cup provides the daily requirement of folate. Split peas and kidney beans serve as great bases for soups and chili.

OMEGA-3 FATTY ACIDS, especially EPA (eicosapentaenoic acid) and DHA (docosahexaenoic acid), are integral to the development of a healthy mother and her baby, since they are not synthesized by the human body. As it directly supports the brain, eyes, and central nervous system, taking 300 mg of DHA daily is hugely beneficial for pregnant and lactating women. Although cold-water fish (salmon, tuna, sardines, anchovies, and herring) are the best sources of EPA and DHA, mercury and other fish toxins remain a realistic concern. As an alternative, reputable fish oil supplements will provide the same benefits but will not taste or smell "fishy."

ORGANIC, FREE-RANGE EGGS are hugely beneficial for expectant mothers. In addition to being protein-rich, eggs are also high in choline, which helps fetal brain development and reduces the risk of birth defects. Uniquely, they are also high in protein while being low in carbohydrates. This helps the body deal with pregnancy-related conditions like gestational diabetes and morning sickness. Not only do eggs help stabilize blood sugar levels but they help keep your energy up during pregnancy. The easily absorbable iron in eggs helps transport oxygen from your lungs to the rest of your body, and ultimately, to your baby.

ROOT VEGETABLES have their good and bad points. The good? Options! Yams, beets, parsnips, turnips, rutabagas, carrots, yucca, kohlrabi, onions, garlic, celery root, horseradish, daikon, turmeric, jicama, Jerusalem artichokes, radishes, and ginger are all classified as root vegetables because they grow underground. As such, they absorb nutrients from the soil and are full of flavor when properly prepared (roasted, steamed, sautéed, or grilled). The bad? They are extremely high in carbohydrates. The ugly? Toxoplasmosis. Contaminated soil can attach to root vegetable skin. Thoroughly washing, scrubbing with a vegetable brush, and peeling the outer skin can help eliminate this exposure without completely removing root vegetables from your diet.

Can I Eat Fish?

To eat or not to eat, that is the question. A common myth is that eating fish during pregnancy is unsafe; however, the iodine, selenium, and omega-3 fatty acids in fish (EPA and DHA) play an important role in your baby's brain and eye development. As the benefits outweigh the potential risks, the real questions pregnant women should ask themselves are, "Am I eating enough fish?" and "Which types of fish are the healthiest for me to eat?" Including fish in your diet helps you vary your protein sources without eating the unnecessary saturated fats associated *with* protein sources. Fish can have different benefits based on where they live and how they are harvested. It's true that certain fish, like shark, swordfish, tilefish, and king mackerel, contain high levels of mercury that can be harmful to you and your developing baby. However, if you follow the specific serving guidelines outlined by the FDA, you will find that you can eat about 12 ounces of *cooked*, low mercury–containing fish (cod, flounder, wild-caught salmon, tilapia, whiting, and scallops) each week during pregnancy.

Fish high in the omega-3 fatty acid DHA (canned or pouch tuna, sardines, anchovies, and trout), boosts the mother's brain health by preventing prenatal and postpartum depression. Getting enough fish and seafood also lowers your baby's risk of childhood obesity and increases heart health.

During the third trimester of pregnancy, as fetal brain development rapidly increases, so do the nutritional requirements, which continue until two years of age.

In Japan, eating raw fish is considered part of sound neonatal nutrition. Yet in the United States, eating raw fish while pregnant is taboo due to the speculative risks of food-borne illnesses, mercury, bacteria, and harmful parasites. Keep in mind that it's really raw mollusks (oysters and clams), and not the fish typically used in sushi, that are responsible for the majority of seafood-related illnesses. Even the fish that are most likely to have parasites, cod and whitefish, are not generally used for sushi. The fatty acids in fish are the ideal nourishment for a growing baby. During pregnancy, choose the restaurants you go to, the preparation methods, and the types of fish you consume wisely, but most important, enjoy your meal.

Anti-Inflammatory Foods

Inflammation begins in your gut. Even though it is a physiologic response to infection, chronic stress, and obesity, inflammation during pregnancy increases a mother's risk of mental illness and interferes with her ability to breastfeed. Addressing the most likely underlying cause of the inflammation, cortisol, the (chronic) stress hormone, is key. Each day, rediscover an activity that relaxes you and brings peace to your space in the world. Whether it is via a massage, a foot soak, or an acupuncture session, allow yourself to unwind. Implementing a stress-reducing, low-impact exercise regimen like walking, prenatal yoga, or aquacise (water aerobics) gets your blood moving in stress-relieving ways that immediately reduce C-reactive protein, the objective measure of inflammation in your body.

As you learn to ease chronic stress and the resulting systemic inflammation, you'll be one step ahead if you are already eating anti-inflammatory foods (fruits, dark leafy greens, nuts, seeds, beans, and foods rich in omega-3 fatty acids). Vegetables in the nightshade family, often erroneously linked to inflammation, represent an allergic reaction rather than an inflammatory response. To really attack that systemic inflammation, add ginger and turmeric to your culinary repertoire while avoiding sugar, artificial sweeteners (no soda or candy), the caffeine in coffee, and alcohol. Over-the-counter medications further contribute to inflammation as they contain synthetic chemicals. Drinking one tablespoon of apple cider vinegar dissolved in water each day reduces inflammation in the digestive system while simultaneously healing the body on the cellular level.

How to Be Pregnant and Vegan

Before getting pregnant, consider how your diet may affect your pregnancy. Many dietary regimens go to extremes, and even if you are able to tolerate them, they may be harmful to your unborn baby. Pregnant women who eat a vegan or vegetarian diet should make sure they're getting enough nutrients for themselves and their unborn child. Talk to your health care provider about ways to properly boost your diet with food options instead of pills, capsules, or tablets. An integrative health provider, nutritionist, dietitian, or clinical herbalist can provide even better guidance to help you stay nourished early on in your pregnancy. Eliminating meat products from your diet means you have to eat enough calories in the form of calorie-dense fruits and vegetables to accommodate your energy needs. You will also need to eat foods from different vegetable protein sources for both you and your developing fetus. Eating a wide array of dried beans (legumes), dried fruits, nuts, seeds, whole grains, peas, lentils, wheat germ, tofu, and other soy products will help you meet your body's demands for iron, zinc, and other trace minerals; however, you'll need to find other sources of calcium, vitamins B2 and B12, and vitamin D. As a vegan or vegetarian, you can absolutely have a healthy pregnancy—just make sure you're eating the right foods and food combinations.

GMOs

The introduction of genetically modified organisms (GMOs) into our food supply is a hotly debated and intensely scrutinized subject. The rationale given for genetically modified foods is twofold: (1) they're resistant to pests, diseases, environmental threats, and herbicides, and (2) they're said to offer improved nutritional value. Unfortunately, more than 80 percent of GMOs contain glyphosate herbicides, which are human carcinogens. Traces of glyphosate have been discovered in the breast milk, urine, and drinking water of American mothers. In addition, some research shows that a large majority of pregnant women and their umbilical cord blood samples contain a pesticide implanted in GMO corn.

CAFFEINE

Caffeine is naturally found in tea (45mg), brewed coffee (95 to 165mg), and chocolate (26mg), and added to energy drinks, cold and flu remedies (65mg), and soda (especially colas, 125mg). Pregnant and breastfeeding women should avoid caffeine as much as possible. Even in small doses, it can cross the placenta and alter your baby's sleep patterns and normal movements. Caffeine isn't only a stimulant, meaning that it increases blood pressure and heart rate, but it's also a diuretic, a substance that increases the frequency of urination, which can lead to dehydration. As described earlier, water is critical; it helps form the placenta, which is how your baby receives nutrients during pregnancy. Water also aids in the formation of the amniotic sac later in your pregnancy. Consequently, pregnancy dehydration can spell bad news, causing complications like neural tube defects, low amniotic fluid, inadequate breast milk production, intrauterine growth restriction, low birth weight, and premature labor and delivery. Even if you feel that you can handle your caffeine intake, it's much harder on your baby. A growing fetus has an immature metabolism that can't manage caffeine well. Studies have shown conflicting results on the amount of caffeine that is acceptable as far as reducing the incidence of miscarriage. As such, there is no real consensus on a "healthy range" for recommended caffeine intake, although 200mg per day, approximately equal to a 12-ounce cup of coffee, is often cited as *safe*. In the meantime, even though researchers are still establishing concrete evidence, avoiding caffeine is your safest bet while pregnant and breastfeeding.

Even though there is no documented research showing any risks in human subjects consuming genetically modified foods, sanctioned experiments conducted in animal studies paint quite a different picture in the toxicology reports. Corn and soy, which are primarily produced to feed livestock, are two of the largest GMO crops in the United States. Our bodies have a challenging time identifying these genetically modified organisms, and they can lead to allergies as well as adverse birth outcomes. For this reason, it's better to eat organic. It can be challenging to opt for food that is always safe and healthy, but the benefits for you and your child are worth it. While it's never a great time to introduce genetically modified organisms into your diet, you should definitely avoid it during pregnancy whenever possible.

How to Eat Pesticide-Free Food

Families commonly spray outdoor pesticides around their home and in their yards to eliminate the threat of garden insects; however, the same chemicals that act on the nervous system of insects also act on your baby's rapidly developing nervous system. It's easy enough for pregnant women to avoid handling or spraying insecticides; it's a little more difficult to ensure pesticide-free food options at all times. Organic foods are sometimes double the price of their conventional counterparts. What's worse, foods labeled "organic" are not all the same.

The Environmental Working Group (EWG) has done the heavy lifting to help you determine how to choose organic and conventional fruits and vegetables. For the budget conscious, its Clean Fifteen list (onion, avocado, sweet corn, pineapple, asparagus, frozen sweet peas, kiwi, cabbage, eggplant, papaya, watermelon, broccoli, cauliflower, cantaloupes, and mushrooms) enables you to buy affordable produce items that are deemed the least con-taminated with pesticides. Similarly, the Dirty Dozen lists the twelve fruits and vegetables (strawberries, spinach, kale, nectarines, apples, grapes, peaches, cherries, pears, tomatoes, celery, and potatoes) that are deemed to be the most contaminated. Whenever possible, choose organic. If you can't choose organic, use a fruit and vegetable wash by mixing 1 cup vin-egar to 4 cups water and 1 tablespoon of lemon juice inside a spray bottle and shake well. Liberally spray the produce, let it sit for about five minutes, then rinse with water, using a vegetable brush if needed. Pat dry with paper towels.

Prenatal Vitamins Unpacked

Birth defects that affect the fetal brain and spine usually occur within the first eight weeks of pregnancy, often before a woman is even aware that she's pregnant. For this reason, women's health professionals and members of the medical community recommend taking prenatal vitamins prior to conception, throughout the pregnancy, and until the conclusion of breastfeeding. Remember, although it can be tempting to rely on prenatal vitamins, they are only designed to supplement a nutritious diet and do not serve as a substitute for any particular food or food group. As much as possible, try to get your necessary vitamins and minerals from the food in your diet.

For women who are chronically stressed, have been taking hormonal birth control for a prolonged period of time, or are vegans, prenatal vitamins help counteract nutritional deficits. In most cases, prenatal vitamins promote a healthy pregnancy by bridging the gap between what is and what could be while creating the optimal environment for fetal development. The obvious benefit of a prenatal vitamin is the nutritional support it offers your growing baby, but its benefits extend to you as well. Prenatal vitamins reduce the risk of harmful conditions like low immunity, postpartum depression, general weakness, and appetite disturbances while reducing annoying symptoms like anemia, fatigue, leg and muscle cramps, and even brain fog. Even though the synthetic nutrients in prenatal vitamins claim to be chemically identical to those found in food-based prenatal vitamins, your body will best use nutrients derived from whole foods.

- **BIOTIN (VITAMIN B7).** Supports the enzymes involved in the metabolism of carbohydrates, fats, and protein and works with the other B vitamins to help release energy from food.

- **CALCIUM.** Dictates the rate of cardiovascular, skeletal, and neurological growth and development. It helps form and maintain healthy teeth and bones for you and your baby.

- **COPPER.** Plays a critical role in iron metabolism and overall blood health. It is essential for red blood cell formation during pregnancy when blood supply doubles.

- **FOLATE/FOLIC ACID (VITAMIN B9).** Prevents birth defects such as neural tube defects and spina bifida. Whole food folic acid supplements are preferable to synthesized folic acid whenever possible.

- **IODINE.** Supports healthy thyroid function, fetal growth, and hearing. A woman needs much more iodine during pregnancy to ensure proper fetal brain development.

IRON. Helps make blood for both you and your baby. It also helps transport blood oxygen throughout the body while supporting fetal growth and development.

MAGNESIUM. Supports healthy blood pressure, reduces preeclampsia, and helps establish a healthy fetal birth weight. It can also help with morning sickness, fatigue, constipation, and gestational diabetes.

NIACIN (VITAMIN B3). Plays a crucial role in metabolism while preventing birth defects and miscarriages. It is essential for fetal brain development, reduces nausea, and improves digestion.

PANTOTHENIC (VITAMIN B5). Helps create hormones and may ease leg cramps. It is essential for the production of cholesterol and helps metabolize carbohydrates, proteins, and fats.

RIBOFLAVIN (VITAMIN B2). Helps the mother produce energy while promoting vision and skin health and reducing preeclampsia risk. Riboflavin is essential for fetal bone, muscle, and nerve development.

THIAMIN (VITAMIN B1). Supports the mother's nervous system and muscle function, helps baby's brain development, and is essential for carbohydrate metabolism, placental function, and growth of the fetus.

VITAMIN A. Helps build baby's immune function, supports visual health, and is important for the development of skin cells and the developing alveoli in your baby's lungs.

VITAMIN B6. Eases pregnancy-related nausea, vomiting, and morning sickness. Along with assisting in fetal brain development and nervous system, vitamin B6 can help form red blood cells.

VITAMIN B12. Promotes the formation of healthy blood cells and helps prevent birth and neurological defects that affect the spine, neural tube, and fetal central nervous system.

VITAMIN C. Boosts your immune system and reduces your risk of iron-deficiency anemia. Vitamin C supports your baby's immune system and helps the fetus absorb iron from food.

CALORIE COUNTING AND CRAVINGS

Although you may feel ravenous during your pregnancy, the idea of "eating for two" is actually misleading—women cannot (and shouldn't) eat twice as much food when they are pregnant. Even though your body absorbs nutrients more efficiently during pregnancy, eating twice the amount of food does not increase your chances of having a healthy baby and actually places you at a higher risk for pregnancy complications. Your baby's development is intimately related to what you eat during pregnancy. Your provider can discuss your specific daily caloric needs based on your pre-pregnancy weight and physical activity; however, if you are within normal or average weight range and are moderately active, you actually don't need any additional calories in the first trimester. In the second trimester, you will need an additional 325 calories a day, the equivalent of a bowl of oatmeal. Even in the third trimester, you'll only need about 500 extra calories a day, the equivalent of about two glasses of milk, a handful of sunflower seeds, or a tuna sandwich.

Depending on your weight gain goals and whether you are overweight or underweight, your daily calories will differ only slightly. To sustain a healthy pregnancy as a mother of multiples, you will need more calories based on the number of babies you are carrying. Despite your cravings for junk food, try to replace calorie-rich, nutrient-poor foods with nutrient-rich snacks like yogurt, nuts, and fresh fruits or vegetables. Strike a balance, allow yourself the occasional indulgence, and try to eat for your blood type. Remember: quality over quantity.

VITAMIN D. Strengthens bones and teeth, helps the body utilize calcium and phosphorus, and decreases the risk of birth complications, such as cesarean section, preeclampsia, preterm birth, and gestational diabetes.

VITAMIN E. Improves maternal blood circulation, which simultaneously improves placental blood circulation. Overall, vitamin E supports delivery of oxygen to the uterus, provides a healthy womb environment, and reduces the risk of miscarriage.

VITAMIN K. Supports healthy bone development and protein formation. It also contributes to blood clotting. Vitamin K taken during the third trimester also helps postpartum wound healing.

ZINC. Supports immune, nerve, and muscle function. The rapid growth and development that takes place in fetal tissue relies heavily on a good supply of zinc.

Supplement Safety

Although prescription and OTC (over-the-counter) drugs are often convenient and readily available, many pregnant women prefer a natural option to provide essential nutrition and symptom relief during pregnancy. Herbal medicine has been successful in managing symptoms ranging from nausea and vomiting to gestational diabetes, preeclampsia prevention, placenta previa management, common colds, low fetal weight, and miscarriage management. Specific herbs (in conjunction with acupuncture) are safe and can be quite effective, especially in older expectant mothers, who often deal with more severe complications.

An integrative approach is key when looking at medicine and herbal remedies during pregnancy. Herbalists are trained in pharmaceutical drug and herbal interactions in ways that most providers are not. For those reasons, pregnant women should not only consult their providers but talk to a licensed and trained herbalist (who may also be an acupuncturist) who is experienced working with women during pregnancy and can offer focused fetal enhancement education. It's important to keep an open dialogue with each of your providers throughout the pregnancy and postpartum periods. Herbal medicine is an effective and safe treatment that generally has no side effects for the mother and the fetus during pregnancy and the postpartum phase. Adding a licensed herbalist to your health care team—in addition to a healthy diet and pharmaceutical regimen—is important before, during, and after pregnancy to make your experience a safe and healthy one for you and your baby.

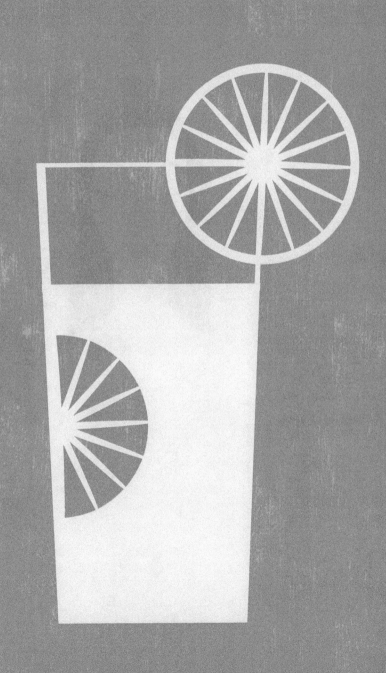

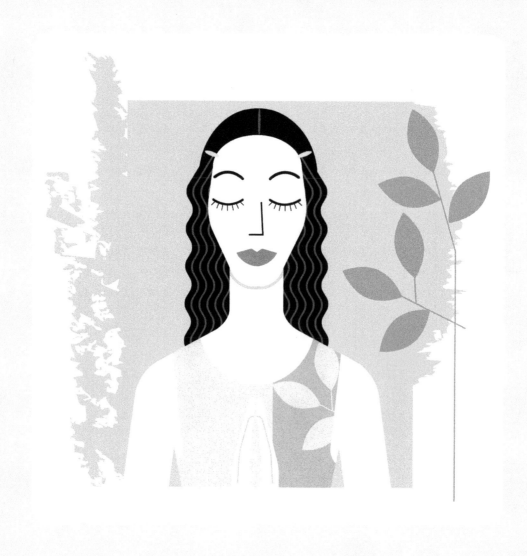

CHAPTER THREE

Mindfulness and Relaxation

Am I eating enough? Will my baby be healthy? I'm afraid of labor. Am I doing enough? Can I really do this? Will I be a good mother? Something doesn't feel right. Do I need to go to the doctor? Am I enough? This is pregnancy anxiety.

Much like parenting, mindfulness is a practice, and you have to practice every day even on the days you do not want to in order to reap the rewards. Proactively incorporating a mindfulness practice into your prenatal care regimen not only protects your own health and well-being but it also protects the health and well-being of your unborn baby by reducing maternal stress and increasing relaxation. Research shows that an established mindfulness regimen helps reduce premature births in high-risk women (low-income and older women) while their babies have higher-than-expected Apgar scores.

The Apgar score, your baby's first test, evaluates your newborn's condition. At one minute and at five minutes someone on your health care team will check the infant's appearance (color), pulse (heart rate), grimace (reflex), activity (muscle tone), and respiration (breathing). A score of 7 to 10 is optimal. If a newborn scores between 4 and 6, they may need resuscitation efforts, including suctioning their airway and administering oxygen. Those who score below 4 will require lifesaving measures.

This chapter will help you develop specific techniques for mental focus that yield positive outcomes. Mindful meditation helps you focus on the physical and emotional aspects of pregnancy that you are experiencing in the present moment without imposing judgment on how you feel. Consistently practicing prenatal mindfulness also yields emotional and physical benefits as you prepare for labor. Research shows that the combination of deep belly breathing and mindfulness meditation can help soften and relax the central nervous system during childbirth, helping alleviate some of the fear of the unknown you may be experiencing. This practice improves the labor experience by contributing to shorter labor and helping decrease the intensity of pain.

Take a Breath

Food consumption and adequate hydration get a great deal of attention during pregnancy, but breathing is just as important. As your uterus enlarges and takes up more space during pregnancy, you may have challenges breathing (even with basic tasks) as it presses against your diaphragm. Your breathing may also be affected by an increase in progesterone, which causes you to breathe in more deeply and often mimics shortness of breath. Progesterone expands your lung capacity, allowing your blood to carry large quantities of oxygen to your baby. Put together, you may feel as if you are working harder to get air. Later in your third trimester, closer to your due date, your baby will begin to descend into your pelvis, and you should start to breathe more easily in preparation for labor and delivery. However, if you have shortness of breath that starts suddenly, is severe, seems to be worsening, or is associated with pain, coughing, wheezing, or heart palpitations, call your provider immediately. For emergencies, call 911, as these symptoms go beyond the normal physiological changes associated with pregnancy.

This section will offer practical advice and exercises for breathing techniques that can reduce nausea and help manage the pain associated with labor and delivery. No matter what, it's always best to talk to your health care provider if you experience shortness of breath, even though it's a common occurrence during pregnancy.

CALM BREATHING FOR NAUSEA AND PAIN

With your eyes closed (or with your eyes open and focused on a physical object), place the tip of your tongue to the roof of your mouth with your lips closed throughout the entire exercise. First empty your lungs with a full exhalation through your nose. Then inhale to a slow count of four (1-2-3-4). Hold your breath through a slow count of seven. Then exhale slowly through your nose to a slow count of eight. Repeat for five cycles or until your symptoms subside. You can also breathe in Peppermint, Lemon, Lavender, Ginger, or Fennel Seed essential oil for slightly faster results.

STOMACH, CHEST, AND SHALLOW BREATHING

To relieve the pressure on your diaphragm, stand up. Raise your arms above your head and then inhale deeply through your nose. Exhaling slowly through the mouth, lower your arms to your sides. Repeat the cycle, rhythmically, this time raising and lowering your head with each inhalation and exhalation, respectively. Focus on the expansion of your chest as fresh air enters your lungs. This breathing technique allows you to bring air into your chest upon inhalation and into your abdomen upon exhalation as your rib cage expands and contracts. As your uterus grows, use this technique whenever breathing becomes difficult.

With your eyes closed and your body relaxed and comfortable, imagine that you are enclosed by a sleep dome that arches over you, providing you with warmth, safety, protection, and comfort. Right now, you are enclosed inside a peaceful, quiet, protective dome that is specifically designed for rest, relaxation, restoration, and deep sleep. With your mind's eye, observe the features of your protective dome (the shape, the size, and the color). Adjust these features until they accommodate your preferences. Outside the shield, nothing exists that needs your attention. You will attend to it tomorrow, when the time is right.

Forest Bathing

Forest bathing, the practice of "taking in the forest" for physical, mental, and spiritual health benefits, started in the 1980s. It is rooted in ancient Japanese reverence to nature and coupled with Shinto and Buddhist traditions. To further conceptualize this practice, consider forest bathing the natural version of putting your phone in airplane mode. The goal is to disconnect from all the distractions while reconnecting to the earth. So often we do not voluntarily take the opportunity to close our laptops, turn off the televisions, and power off our phones in order to slow down and take in our natural surroundings. By intentionally and deliberately looking around, smelling the air, listening to the whisper of the breeze and animals, and grounding ourselves in the natural environment of the earth, forest bathing induces relaxation; lowers blood pressure; boosts mood, immunity, and energy; soothes sore muscles; and naturally aids in sleep.

A forest that is heavily wooded with conifer trees (cedars, Douglas firs, cypresses, pines, hemlocks, redwoods, and spruces) is best, but any heavily wooded area will do. Stay focused on relaxation by forest bathing in an ideal location with comfortable temperature and minimal noise and distractions. Even if you are not able to take advantage of Mother Nature's bounty, you can utilize essential oils (Cypress, Pine, Juniper, Cedarwood, and Fir) to re-create the experience in your local environment. Using a diffuser to disseminate the scent of conifer coupled with frankincense promotes an anti-inflammatory response.

Affirmations and Visualizations

If you're feeling nervous about pregnancy, you may find yourself talking (and thinking) about it in ways that project negative, anxious, and stressful emotions. You may do this without even being aware of it. Unconsciously, though, these self-defeating statements can have a negative effect on how you cope with and relate to yourself during pregnancy, labor, and the post-partum breastfeeding stage. Using affirmations to promote positive thinking is a common prenatal practice that can ease anxiety and fear. Since your thoughts and emotions directly affect your unborn baby's development, you'll want to make sure you are doing all you can to help your baby grow, develop, and flourish.

Repeated daily affirmations can help women who are having anxious thoughts turn those negative feelings into positive ones. Like a positive feedback loop, this newfound affirmative willingness rewires and further strengthens the brain to stimulate positive feelings. Putting these positive messages on notes around the house, in the car, and in your office helps reinforce confidence and readiness. Eventually, these simple notes will become ingrained personal beliefs. To be clear, affirmations do not guarantee specific pregnancy and birth outcomes, but they can reduce stress and anxiety by making it easier to relax. Writing your own affirmations helps you visualize the statements as truth. Practicing and remembering key affirmations is one of the best things you can do for yourself, your pregnancy, and your unborn child, as they will help you have a calmer pregnancy that you can truly enjoy.

AFFIRMATIONS

Once you are in a comfortable position with your hands resting on your womb, take a slow, deep breath and repeat the following positive affirmations to yourself (both silently and out loud):

I am excitedly welcoming the daily visual changes in my pregnant body because these changes reflect the healthy growth and development of my unborn child.

My mind, body, and spirit are open to the challenges of motherhood and I will graciously accept these challenges with gratitude and a loving heart.

My pregnant body is divinely designed and I am perfectly equipped to labor and give birth comfortably, easily, peacefully, joyfully, and in my natural ability.

My baby senses the peace I feel, and will find the perfect position and be born at the perfect time, the true birthday.

My body trusts my baby and accepts that my pregnancy will end with the safe birth of a beautifully healthy baby who is already loved.

My productive labor contractions are preparing me for a safe and effortless birthing experience that will bring my baby into my arms, and I am ready.

Breastfeeding is one of my most important jobs as a mother and I will remain relaxed so that I make plenty of milk for my baby.

I know how to take care of myself during this pregnancy because I am bringing a perfectly healthy, whole, and strong child into this world.

My body knows how to nourish my baby adequately so that my unborn child can healthily grow and develop in the safety of my womb.

I am a strong, courageous woman and a confidently devoted mother who will make the right decisions for my baby throughout my pregnancy, labor, and delivery.

VISUALIZATIONS

1. With both of your hands on your womb, gently cradle your baby. Observe the sensations you feel under your fingertips and beneath your hands. Do you feel warmth? Is your baby moving? How are they positioned? Breathe slowly, in and out. If your mind wanders off, breathe deeper into your womb. If a negative thought arises, let it float away, as if floating down a stream. Do this for at least five minutes each day, gradually adding more time each week as you feel comfortable.

2. With your eyes closed, inhale and exhale deeply and slowly. Picture your favorite place to relax. Now picture yourself relaxing in this place. Observe. Describe the temperature. How do you feel? What do you see? Let the colors envelop you. Are you alone? Who is there with you? Your baby? Do you see animals? Are there plants or trees? What music do you hear? Do you hear any sounds? What are they? What does it smell like? Once you have observed everything, bid this place farewell, and gently open your eyes, reveling in your calm.

3. Close your eyes, breathing deeply as you allow every single part of your body, from your forehead to your toes, to feel light. Relax into a comfortable position as you prepare to journey into your womb. As if you had x-ray vision, look into your womb. What do you see? What do you notice about your unborn child? Is your baby floating? Are you able to see its face? Which side of your body are they on? Are they angled to the right or the left? Are they sucking their thumb? Enjoy being with your baby in this way.

4. In your preferred meditation position, close your eyes and relax inward. Placing your hands on your womb, feel your skin. Feel the warmth beneath your hands. Feel the firm places on your abdomen and the soft places underneath your hands. Bring your attention to your unborn baby. Make a wish for them. What do you desire for your baby? Make a wish for your baby's health and for their life. Allow yourself to thoroughly enjoy this experience before opening your eyes.

5. Close your eyes and get comfortable in the meditative position of your choosing. Put your hands underneath your womb as you direct light, love, and warmth to your baby. Softly connect your breath to your baby. With each breath, guide clear oxygen to your baby. With each inhale, breathe in the oxygen that your baby needs. Your baby needs you to take care of them, so be kind to yourself. You are enough. You are the perfect mom for them. Inhale deeply. Exhale slowly. Inhale peace. Exhale love. As you carry this feeling of peace with you, gently open your eyes.

Start Exercising

In most cases, exercise is safe during pregnancy. If you are healthy and your pregnancy is low risk, you may continue your pre-pregnancy exercise regimen. If you were not active prior to pregnancy, you can take this opportunity to begin regular physical activity. Exercise helps you stay in shape during pregnancy and strengthens you for the work of labor and delivery. Physical activity does not increase your risk of miscarriage or early delivery; however, you should discuss your exercise regimen with your health care team at each prenatal visit. Maintaining a regular exercise schedule throughout your pregnancy will help you stay healthy and energized while benefiting your posture and decreasing fatigue. Exercise can also prevent gestational diabetes and alleviate stress.

If you have never regularly exercised, you can safely begin walking during pregnancy. Walking is a great exercise for beginners, as it is low impact while providing moderate aerobic conditioning. Swimming, water aerobics, and cycling are also sound alternatives. With each workout, remember to warm up, stretch, and cool down while drinking plenty of fluids to stay hydrated. The American College of Obstetricians and Gynecologists recommends at least 30 minutes of moderate exercise per day at least four days a week.

YOGA

Joining a prenatal yoga class will help you breathe and relax. As you adjust to the physical demands of pregnancy and prepare for labor and delivery, yoga calms both the mind and body, which alleviates physical and emotional stress. Avoid any asanas (poses) that require lying on your back, as they reduce blood flow to the uterus. In addition, avoid Bikram yoga ("hot" yoga) because overheating endangers the health of your developing baby. Even in a prenatal yoga class, pay attention to your body and stop if you feel uncomfortable. Modify each pose as your body changes.

SWIMMING

Swimming is a safe pregnancy exercise; however, if swimming is a new activity for you, consult with your provider before you begin. Swimming helps improve circulation, increase muscle tone, build endurance, and promote sleep.

Swimming is a uniquely beneficial exercise in pregnancy because the water helps support your pregnancy weight—which can be a welcome reprieve for pregnancy aches and pains. Be mindful to alternate your strokes. Spend equal time swimming on your front, floating on your back, and gently kicking your legs to give yourself a comprehensive workout. Start slowly and gradually extend your session to 30 minutes.

CARDIO

All pregnant women should avoid any cardiovascular exercise that puts them at risk for falls or collisions. Prioritizing strength workouts during pregnancy is key because hormones and a continually growing midsection leave you moderately unstable. However, cardiovascular activity throughout pregnancy is still important. You'll need to modify your workouts and be sure to warm up and cool down afterward, no matter which cardiovascular activity you choose. Be sure to stretch after working out when your muscles, ligaments, and tendons are warm and loose. Remember to stay hydrated all throughout the workout and listen to your body by taking breaks as needed.

A Good Night's Sleep

Sleep is the final piece of the puzzle when charting a course of natural health during pregnancy. Now is the time to prioritize sleep, to come up with an effective strategy for managing sleep challenges, and to take sleep seriously. According to The American Journal of Obstetrics and Gynecology, women who slept less than 6 hours at night had longer labors and were 4.5 times more likely to have cesarean deliveries. They recommend 8 hours of sleep per night. For many pregnant women, getting 8 to 10 hours of sleep each night becomes increasingly difficult the further along they are in their pregnancy. The amount of sleep you get (or don't get) during pregnancy affects you and your baby and also affects your labor and delivery.

When you become pregnant, fatigue is one of the first symptoms you notice due to the ever-increasing size of the fetus, which can make it difficult to find a comfortable sleeping position. Being a habitual back or stomach sleeper may also prove to be a challenge since providers recommend sleeping on your side in order to maintain proper blood flow and oxygenation to the placenta. In addition, rising progesterone levels can cause excessive daytime sleepiness, especially in the first trimester. For first time mothers, insomnia is also a real concern due to emotional changes, anxiety about labor and delivery, balancing work and home life, and the changing relationship with their partner.

THE FIVE MOST COMMON SLEEP PROBLEMS

1. SIDE SLEEPING is uncomfortable, especially if you are accustomed to another position. It is, however, the position most beneficial for your unborn child.

2. RESTLESSNESS AND ANXIETY can interrupt sleep to the point of full-blown insomnia. Practice your calming techniques and relaxation breathing to get back to sleep.

3. HEARTBURN, CONSTIPATION, AND INDIGESTION will continue to worsen into the third trimester as the growing uterus presses against the stomach and the large intestine.

4. LEG CRAMPS AND BACKACHES result from the extra pregnancy weight you are carrying and the simultaneous loosening of ligaments through-out the body.

5. FREQUENT URINATION results in more trips to the bathroom at night as the kidneys are filtering more blood and the uterus continues to grow.

TEN TIPS FOR BETTER SLEEP

1. **ELIMINATE FLUIDS AT NIGHT.** In order to stay hydrated enough during pregnancy, you may need to redistribute the total amount of liquid you consume throughout the day.

2. **SLEEP ON YOUR LEFT SIDE.** Providers recommend that expectant mothers sleep on their left side to increase blood flow to the placenta and fetus.

3. **EXERCISE REGULARLY.** Consistently exercising at least 30 minutes a day improves circulation, mood, and sleep quality. No vigorous exercise should be done close to bedtime.

4. **MAINTAIN A REGULAR SLEEP CYCLE.** *Prioritizing* sleep is the key to sleeping. Establish a consistent sleep/wake schedule all week to feel more energized throughout the day.

5. **GO TO BED WITH A CLEAR HEAD.** Empty yourself of worries, stress, and anxious thoughts before bed by journaling your thoughts in a night-stand notebook.

6. **AVOID SPICY FOODS AND HEAVY MEALS BEFORE BEDTIME.** Eating spicy foods before bedtime causes heartburn. Eating heavy meals before bedtime can cause digestive issues.

7. **WHEN HAVING TROUBLE SLEEPING, GET OUT OF BED.** Do not lie in bed waiting to fall asleep. Do another relaxing activity before returning to bed.

8. **USE PILLOWS.** Pregnancy pillows increase comfort by reducing back pain. Placing pillows between your knees, under your abdomen, and behind your back can also alleviate pain.

9. **COOL DOWN.** Lower the thermostat in the bedroom and leave a blanket at the foot of the bed to pull up if you feel chilly.

10. **TAKE NAPS DURING THE DAY.** Napping while pregnant is beneficial. Be sure to limit naps to 20 to 30 minutes and don't nap close to bedtime.

Sleep Aids

Some women have trouble getting a good night's sleep even with sound sleep practices. Combatting insomnia in pursuit of quality sleep can feel like a Herculean task. If you continue to wake up not feeling well-rested, you may need extra help to nod off naturally. Every expectant woman has specific needs in terms of achieving comfortable, quality, uninterrupted sleep prior to her baby's arrival. For every trimester, customary sleep position, temperature, and potential environmental disturbance, there is a natural sleep aid (maternity pillows, ergonomic pregnancy pillows, wedges, and white noise sound machines) that addresses and caters to your need for quality, uninterrupted sleep. The following remedies can also be helpful.

CHAMOMILE AND VALERIAN ROOT TEAS

Herbal teas, Western and Chinese remedies alike, have been used as natural sleep remedies for years. Chamomile tea contains the antioxidant apigenin, which helps initiate sleep. Valerian root tea improves overall sleep quality by shortening the time it takes to fall asleep and decreasing the number of sleep interruptions.

MELATONIN

Multifunctional melatonin-infused creams not only help with sleep but also soothe the body and enhance skin hydration. As amazing as this sounds, melatonin is not for everyone. As with all supplements, consult with your provider before applying melatonin to your skin or consuming it as a supplement.

MAGNESIUM

Coupled with melatonin, magnesium helps manage sleep by regulating the neurotransmitters that calm the nervous system. Studies have also shown that magnesium encourages deeper, more replenishing sleep. Be sure to talk to your provider about the correct dosage, since excess magnesium may cause diarrhea.

PILLOWS

Ergonomic maternity pillows (U-shaped pillows, C-shaped pillows, wedges, and inflatable varieties) are designed for each trimester and customary sleep position. Full body pillows are specifically designed to support the back and hips while aligning your body properly. There are different varieties of maternity pillows, each with unique shapes and benefits, so you may need to check out a few to find the one that works best for you.

WHITE NOISE MACHINES

Sometimes annoying environmental stimuli can keep you awake at night. Passing cars, sirens, and the natural nighttime noises in your house can exacerbate sleep challenges. White noise machines block out exterior noises using different pitches of white noise or calming nature sounds. Some women find that they also soothe anxiety.

COOLING AIDS

For many pregnant women, overheating and temperature discomfort are the main reasons they cannot obtain quality, uninterrupted sleep. They experience major challenges staying cool during the summer months and even at night throughout the year. Pregnancy pillows, specifically designed to help sleep, often make matters worse. Consider upgrading your sheets to light-colored, 100 percent cotton or linen sheets instead of silk or satin varieties that trap heat when they cling to your body. If air-conditioning is challenging or simply not ideal for you, you can always make your own. Fill a tray with ice and place it directly in front of a fan. As the ice evaporates, the cooler air will be spread around the room you're in.

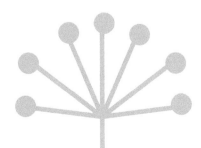

OXYTOCIN: THE LOVE HORMONE

Oxytocin is intimately associated with feelings of empathy, trust, and relationship-building. Both hugging and sexual activity stimulate the release of oxytocin, and there seems to be a positive correlation between oxytocin concentration and the intensity of the mother's orgasm. Oxytocin, a naturally occurring hormone, also plays an intimate role in childbirth and breastfeeding. During childbirth, oxytocin signals the uterus to contract, which starts labor. In the postpartum stage, oxytocin reduces bleeding after childbirth and is responsible for helping the uterus return to its pre-pregnancy size. During breastfeeding, when a baby latches on to its mother's breast, the action triggers a release of oxytocin, which signals the body's milk letdown for the baby.

Oxytocin has positive effects on the mother-child bond as well. Studies have shown that mothers with higher oxytocin levels are more likely to display affectionate parenting behaviors such as periodic "checking-in" on the baby, affectionate touching, singing and speaking to the baby in loving ways, and caring grooming and bathing behaviors. Similarly, babies who receive this type of caring parenting experience a reciprocal boost of oxytocin, which encourages them to seek more contact with their mother (or primary caregiver), further strengthening this bond.

Try the following behaviors to boost oxytocin in the brain:

- Talking to your unborn baby and repeatedly singing them the same songs are great for oxytocin release; the songs will also soothe your baby after birth.

- Nesting, decorating, setting up your baby's nursery, and gathering baby clothes in your room are precursor activities to affectionate and caring motherhood.

- Taking time to consider, with intention, what you will enjoy doing with your child at key milestones in their life can help you feel welcoming and loving toward your baby.

- Telling your unborn child how much you lovingly adore them sets the foundation for a loving relationship with your child.

- Dancing prepares your body for labor. Move your hips in figure eights, focusing on the movements that feel good. Let your body be your guide.

- Engaging in skin-to-skin contact with your partner or a loved one raises your oxytocin levels. This will help you discover the birth instincts that will guide you through delivery.

- Kissing your romantic partner not only raises your oxytocin levels, but it will also help open your birth canal. In early labor, I encourage a lot of kissing while labor progresses. The mouth and throat are hardwired to your pelvic floor and birth canal, so by opening the mouth and throat you are directly opening the pelvic floor muscles and the birth canal.

- Eating dates four to six weeks before your due date brings you benefits from their oxytocin-like effects. Dates help ripen the cervix and increase tolerance to pain.

- Massaging your nipples or stimulating them through your baby's breastfeeding latch triggers the release of oxytocin. If labor slows down, nipple stimulation gets the oxytocin flowing again. The release of oxytocin also relaxes you and the baby.

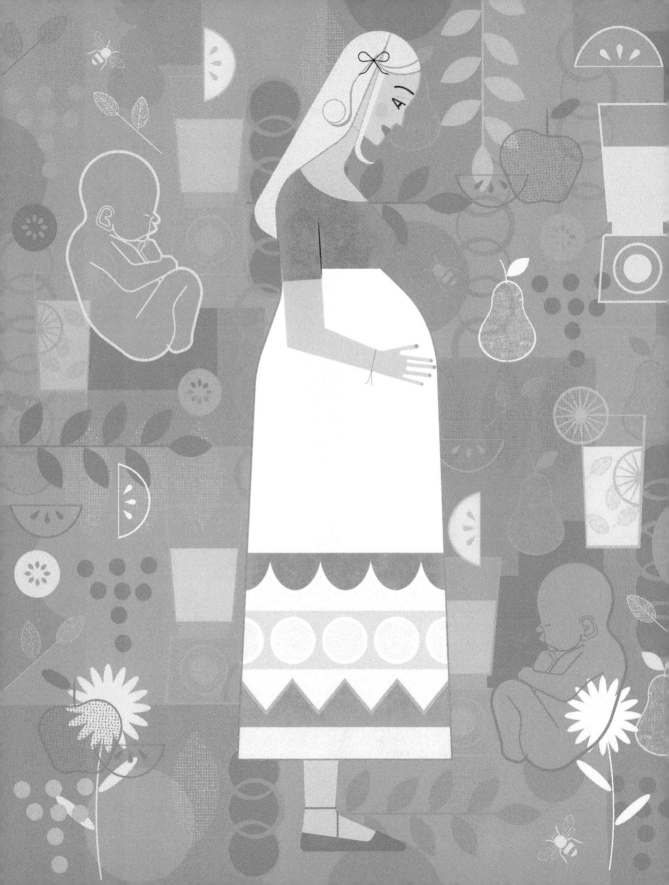

Part Two

A WHOLE, HEALTHY PREGNANCY

Congratulations! You have decided to provide your baby with a firm foundation based on health and wellness. Keep in mind, though, that your baby does not come into this world without you. This decision is about the pair, healthy mother and baby.

Now that you have a baseline for establishing healthy habits during your pregnancy, you can continue pondering the details of what an unadulterated pregnancy means to *you*. For every expectant mother, this aspect of the book (and your life) will be different. There is no wrong approach. Conception, pregnancy, and delivery are natural life experiences. Even though your body is impeccably designed for this work (yes, *work*), like any job or task worth doing, bringing your baby into this world requires intentional preparation coupled with the strength and stamina necessary to sustain a healthy, flourishing pregnancy.

The chapters in this section focus on each trimester. In each chapter, you will find key milestones for you and your baby, including checklists, insights into organizing your birth plan and baby registry, and information regarding the *art* and *science* of pregnancy. Each chapter will close with recipes and essential oil formulas that address trimester-specific challenges.

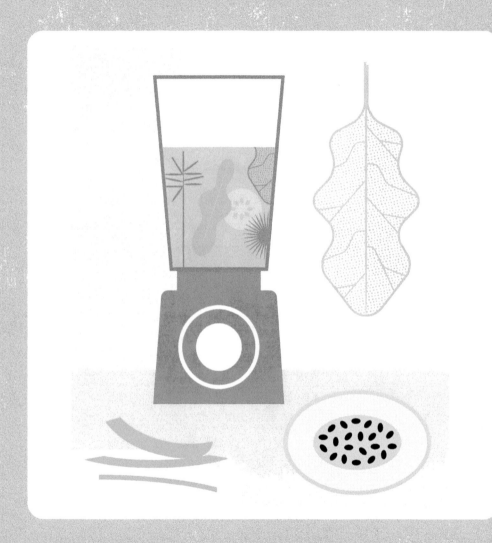

CHAPTER FOUR

The First Trimester

Your first trimester extends from week 1 to week 13. Most people refer to pregnancy in terms of months; however, your health care provider will calculate your pregnancy in weeks based on the start of your last menstrual period (if your periods are regular). If you have missed a period and have taken a home pregnancy test with a positive result, then you are already at least two weeks pregnant. You might have been well into this trimester before you even knew you were pregnant. This is the beginning of your pregnancy journey and it may even be the most difficult trimester for you. During the first four weeks, you will not *look* pregnant, though you'll probably start to feel pregnant with tender breasts and minor fatigue. Weeks 5 to 8 bring about some subtle changes that you may barely recognize or might merely consider annoying (frequent trips to the bathroom, bloat, extra saliva, and increasing fatigue) more than actual challenges. Exhaustion coupled with nausea and vomiting, the hallmarks of morning sickness, may accompany the last weeks of the first trimester, but hearing the beautiful first sounds of your baby's heartbeat will make it all worthwhile.

Wherever you are in your pregnancy, you are exactly where you need to be. Pause. Take a deep breath. Relax. You are beginning one of the most gratifying journeys of your life. This chapter (and all the others) is full of advice that will make your first trimester easier and will help make the transition between trimesters much smoother.

How's My Baby?

By the end of the first four weeks of pregnancy, your baby is an embryo shaped like a tadpole and smaller than a grain of rice. Even though your embryo does not quite resemble a human being yet, the shape of the head (including a basic brain in its earliest stage of development) is beginning to mature; there is even an opening where the mouth will be soon. The heart is in the early stages of development and has begun pumping. Even though your baby is still considered an embryo at the end of week 8, it is about an inch long and will soon start to resemble a baby. Arms, feet, fingers, and toes are visible, yet they are still in the developmental stage. There will be imperceptible movements in your womb while the placenta forms.

During the last weeks of the first trimester, your baby becomes a fetus and is about three inches long. It will begin to look, well, human as the eyes move closer together to the front and the ears arrange themselves to the side of the head. Soft nails begin to cover the fingers and toes. At this point your baby is about the size of an apple and weighs a little more than an ounce. A disproportionate head, which makes up about one-third of the body length, is now supported by a distinguishable neck. If you want to know the sex of your baby, you can find out because external genitalia will have developed enough to make this distinction by the end of the first trimester.

How Am I?

During the first four weeks of your pregnancy, people will not notice that you are pregnant. You, on the other hand, will begin to notice that your breasts may feel fuller and your lower abdomen may often feel bloated. You might also have some light queasiness accompanied by a hypersensitivity to certain scents. Emotionally, PMS-like symptoms (mood swings, irritability, and weepiness) can arise, too. By the end of week eight, even though you still may not *feel* pregnant, your uterus will be the size of a grapefruit (pre-pregnancy, it is the size of your fist).

You still may not appear to be pregnant to other people; however, your clothes will begin to feel snug and more uncomfortable around your waist. You may start having more food cravings and aversions around this time and you may also begin to experience constipation and some minor white vaginal discharge. You may have some dizzy spells and occasional headaches. Your fuller breasts may also warrant a new bra.

Your emotions will also change, ranging from disbelief to elation, including feelings of fear. As the first trimester ends, a paradoxical sense of calm will come over you. Your large grapefruit-size uterus can be felt right above your pubic bone now. Your waistline will begin to disappear and you'll start regaining your appetite as morning sickness subsides. As your blood supply increases, you will become aware of visible veins on your legs and abdomen. Throughout this trimester, if you experience any bleeding, call your provider immediately.

How's My Pregnancy?

Prenatal care is necessary for the optimal growth and development of your baby. Throughout your pregnancy, there should be a consistent, open dialogue with your provider, even between appointments. Exercise is important for you, and regardless of your pre-pregnancy exercise habits, finding the right pregnancy workout program for you and discussing it with your provider is also important. At your first few appointments, your provider will perform laboratory tests (blood work, urinalysis and culture, and tests for sexually transmitted diseases) and a pelvic examination (including a Pap smear), and may also test for your blood type. By the latter part of the first trimester, you and your baby will have reached a pivotal developmental milestone, as the risk of miscarriage drops drastically. At this point in your pregnancy, your provider may recommend chorionic villus sampling (CVS) versus amniocentesis if she suspects genetic abnormalities such as Down syndrome, Tay-Sachs disease, sickle cell anemia, or cystic fibrosis in your fetus. This prenatal diagnostic test, conducted when there is a family history of disease or when the parents are known carriers, uses a small tissue sample from finger-like projections of the placenta to detect chromosomal abnormalities. As the first trimester ends, you will have a sonogram to further evaluate your pregnancy. This may be an opportunity for you to hear your baby's heartbeat and obtain the first predelivery picture of them.

In addition to the clinical aspects of pregnancy, now is the ideal time to start thinking about the financial part. Changes in cost, insurance coverage, benefits, and hospital accommodations will all factor into your decision-making process.

The Aches and Pains

Pregnancy can be filled with amazing moments and experiences . . . and it can also be filled with a slew of annoying symptoms. Many of these symptoms you'll discuss with your provider, whereas some you will choose to share with your friends. Other symptoms, common though they are, will be rather embarrassing, and you will just as easily want to forget them. As your uterus changes with the size of your growing baby, other parts of your body will also change. Although some of these changes are due to the pregnancy hormones, there are some additional physical and emotional changes that accompany the growth of your baby. Every woman and every pregnancy is different, and there are no *universal* pregnancy symptoms. If there's anything you're unsure about, talk to your provider. Understanding and preparing for these changes will help you manage them better if (and when) they arise.

MORNING SICKNESS

Nausea (with or without vomiting), collectively known as morning sickness, is common during the first trimester. However, feeling nauseous isn't guaranteed. In fact, the phrase "morning sickness" is a misnomer, because nausea and vomiting can occur at any point in the day, not just in the morning. Although there are a lot of theories as to why morning sickness occurs, your rapidly increasing pregnancy hormones, hCG and estrogen, combined with temporarily inefficient digestion are the main culprits. The good news? Even if you vomit so often that you lose weight during your first trimester, you are not harming your baby. Although there is no instant cure for morning sickness, there are ways to minimize its effects as you wait for the first trimester to pass. Since nausea is most likely to strike when you have an empty stomach, even before getting out of bed, start the day off by eating a handful of dry cereal, homemade trail mix, crackers, or rice cakes that you keep on your nightstand. Eating light, high-protein snacks and complex carbohydrates frequently throughout the day will help you fend off the queasiness. In addition to changing your diet, getting acupuncture from a licensed acupuncturist who specializes in treating pregnant women can also be beneficial.

SPOTTING, BLEEDING, AND DISCHARGE

Bleeding or spotting early on during your pregnancy is an ominous symptom that might cause some concern. You may wonder about the viability of your pregnancy and the possibility of a miscarriage. However, bleeding at some point during your first trimester is actually not that unusual. Slight spotting or discharge doesn't have to be an emergency situation. If you notice any spotting or bleeding, regardless of the amount, contact your provider for guidance. Be sure to include as many details as possible, including any corresponding symptoms, even if they seem trivial.

SORE BREASTS

Tender, swollen breasts are often one of the cardinal signs of pregnancy (especially if your menstrual period does not begin as expected). Moving into the second trimester, you may find that your slightly tender breasts have become painfully swollen and enlarged. Though your partner may be excited about this change, you'll need to clearly communicate your pain and discomfort so that you are not resenting your partner while also suffering in silence. Toward the end of the first trimester, the tenderness will ease up a bit. The enlargement and sensitivity, however, may prove to heighten your sexual interactions.

CONSTIPATION

At some point in your pregnancy, constipation (hard-to-pass stools or irregular bowel movements) accompanied with bloating, gas, and pain will probably appear. Progesterone, which increases in your body during pregnancy, slows digestion, and if you're taking iron supplements you may also be more prone to constipation. Drinking plenty of water (and prune juice) will help you avoid constipation, along with eating high-fiber foods like beans and bran cereal. Body movement also helps, so get out there and go for a walk. Despite the discomfort, try not to strain while going to the bathroom, since doing so may lead to hemorrhoids. Also, do not use commercial laxatives without talking to your provider first.

FATIGUE

During early pregnancy, you are going to experience some fatigue as your body works to support the new life growing within you. Progesterone, again, plays a leading role here. You can combat fatigue by making a point of sleeping more than you usually did before pregnancy. A healthy diet and consistent exercise will also help boost your energy levels. Let the dishes wait. Order your groceries online and have them delivered. Enjoy takeout. If the task is not essential, allow someone else to take care of it. Take the opportunity to pamper yourself by spending an evening with your feet up, taking a midafternoon nap, or reading a leisure book. As difficult as it might be to do, take people up on their offers and allow them to take care of you (even if it's something you can do for yourself).

FREQUENT URINATION

As the uterus grows throughout pregnancy, it places pressure on the bladder. If you haven't already done so, curb your intake of caffeine by limiting coffee, tea, and cola. These drinks not only increase urination but they also exacerbate fatigue. If your sleep is interrupted by trips to the bathroom, stay away from beverages of any kind within two hours of bedtime (but don't limit drinks during the day). Kegel exercises can also help by strengthening the pelvic floor muscles and improving bladder control, which eliminates leaks when you cough or sneeze (yes, this happens). To make sure that you are completely emptying your bladder, try leaning forward when you are urinating.

MOODINESS

Peaking pregnancy hormones may cause uncontrollable mood swings. Dips in blood sugar can lead to mood crashes, so keep your blood sugar level on target by eating complex carbohydrates and protein, such as muffins, cheese, turkey, chicken, and nuts. Similarly, avoid sugar and caffeine, since those spike glucose levels. And don't forget to exercise! Movement releases endorphins, keeping your mood positive (and yes, sex *is* exercise). When possible, bask in the sunshine to lighten your mood. Rest and relax to counteract the fatigue and stress, which make mood swings more pronounced. Your partner may need help understanding what is going on. Talk openly and speak candidly about what you need, what helps, and what doesn't.

WEIGHT GAIN

Regardless of your pre-pregnancy weight, now is not the time to drastically change your diet. Some women gain two to four (permanent) pounds with each pregnancy, whereas some gain much more: Still others do not put on any permanent weight. Weight gain is woman-specific and pregnancy-specific. With cravings, you may eat foods that are not optimal, which can increase weight gain. Similarly, morning sickness can kill your appetite, causing you to gain less weight. The key to gaining the appropriate amount of weight is a healthy diet and consistent exercise. Gaining the correct amount of weight at the right pace will enable you to lose your baby weight within three to six months after delivery and possibly sooner, especially if you choose to breastfeed.

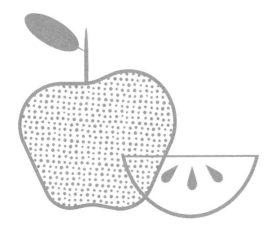

A Green Registry Checklist

In preparation for baby's arrival, organizing an eco-registry filled with organic and renewable items is an ideal task to tackle during the first trimester. You will feel at ease selecting earth-friendly options that not only align with a "green" pregnancy but also protect your newborn in the process. While each of the items listed is important, every family has a budget. Prioritize with the top of the list and work your way down.

- ☐ CAR SEAT. Chemical-free fabric, ergonomic design, no flame-retardant chemicals added

- ☐ CLOTHING. Gender-neutral, organic cotton that is breathable and keeps baby cool

- ☐ CLOTH DIAPERS AND REUSABLE SWIM DIAPERS. Made from biodegradable materials or compostable inserts with adjustable snaps

- ☐ SWADDLE/RECEIVING BLANKET. Natural cotton, breathable, lightweight, warm, doubles as toddler playmat

- ☐ SKIN CARE. Products free from parabens, dyes, perfumes, phthalates, chlorine, and sodium laureth sulfate

- ☐ COCONUT OIL. Used for diaper rash instead of diaper cream or lanolin

- ☐ CLOTH WIPES. A natural extension of cloth diapers, from organically grown products

- ☐ BRUSH AND COMB. Wooden, natural bristles for cradle cap, massages and to stimulate the scalp

- ☐ CARRIER WRAP. Breathable, naturally antibacterial bamboo fibers with optional ultraviolet protection feature

- ☐ CARRIER. Organic cotton, ergonomically designed for baby with multiple carrier positions

- ☐ DISPOSABLE DIAPERS. Plant-based layers (citrus and chlorophyll), no chlorine, no bleach

- ☐ **STROLLER.** Lightweight, eco-conscious manufacturing, retractable canopy, made from recyclable materials

- ☐ **DIAPER BAG.** 100 percent polyurethane "vegan" leather, no PVC, storage, insulated pockets

- ☐ **GLASS BOTTLES.** Thermal shock-resistant glass, dishwasher safe, free from BPA and phthalates

- ☐ **CHANGING PAD.** Organic cotton, waterproof cover, safety straps, low chemical emissions

- ☐ **PROTECTIVE PILLOW COVERS.** Organic bamboo, allergen and dust mite barrier, 100 percent cotton

- ☐ **LOUNGER/RECLINER.** Organic, compostable, doubles as a co-sleeping pillow and infant lounger

- ☐ **CRIB.** Nontoxic finish, no lead, no phthalates, sustainable wood, convertible

- ☐ **CRIB SHEETS.** 100 percent pure organic cotton, super soft, durable, breathable

- ☐ **MATTRESS AND MATTRESS PADS.** Free from volatile organic compounds (VOCs) like formaldehyde, benzene, and toluene

- ☐ **TEETHER.** Made from food-grade materials, free from BPA, phthalates, PVC, and latex

- ☐ **HIGH CHAIR.** Easy-to-clean, adjustable height, plant-based lacquer, renewable materials, nontoxic finish

- ☐ **PLASTIC BOTTLES.** Recyclable, silicone nipple, no BPA, phthalates, lead, PET, or PVC

- ☐ **ACTIVITY GYM.** 100 percent wood, chemical-free, nontoxic, eco-friendly, handmade organic cotton materials

- ☐ **NURSERY FURNITURE.** Sustainably grown and responsibly harvested materials

ULTRASOUNDS ARE SAFER
THAN THE ALTERNATIVE

Risk accompanies all medical procedures. Some women may worry about the safety of ultrasounds, even though there is not enough scientific consensus to give any reason for concern. Most medical researchers agree that ultrasound exams, when conducted by a physician or trained professional, do not pose any significant risk to the mother or the baby. Ultrasound technology provides information about fetal well-being, including fetal age and growth, number of fetuses, location of the placenta, fetal position, movement, breathing, heart rate, amount of amniotic fluid in the uterus, the length of the cervix, and some birth defects.

By using transducers, ultrasounds direct sound wave energy, not radiation, into the body. The sound waves echo off the fetus and then transform into a visual representation of the fetus that can be seen on a screen. Ultrasound testing gives the provider and the pregnant woman reassurance about the pregnancy and overall fetal condition. However, you do have options (and some alternatives) to this kind of testing. Ultrasounds that show a three- or four-dimensional image, while aesthetically pleasing, are not medically necessary and can be avoided. Unless your provider suspects an ectopic pregnancy, ultrasounds prior to week 12 are also unnecessary to confirm pregnancy. A simple blood test will confirm pregnancy during this time period. Although not having an ultrasound throughout your pregnancy is ill-advised, you do not have to accept each ultrasound that is offered to you. If your provider recommends an ultrasound and you have concerns, don't hesitate to express them.

Recipes for the First Trimester

PEACHES AND CREAM NO-COOK OVERNIGHT OATS

LIGHT BITE, QUICK AND EASY

SERVES 1 / PREP TIME: 5 MINUTES

Overnight oats are a great way to prep your breakfast ahead of time. They are a simple, healthy grab-and-go option and often work well for women in their first trimester of pregnancy who want something on the lighter side. You can have them cold if warm foods do not appeal to you.

½ cup rolled oats

⅓ cup plain, unsweetened yogurt (use almond or cashew milk yogurt if avoiding dairy)

¼ cup unsweetened almond milk

1 teaspoon vanilla extract

1 teaspoon maple syrup

2 teaspoons chia seeds

½ peach, sliced (or 4 slices canned peaches in their own juice)

1. In a small bowl or mason jar, combine the oats, yogurt, almond milk, vanilla extract, maple syrup, and chia seeds. Mix well.
2. Add sliced peaches on top.
3. Cover, let sit overnight, and enjoy in the morning.

PER SERVING: Calories: 312; Total fat: 7g; Saturated fat: 1g; Cholesterol: 5mg; Sodium: 103mg; Carbohydrates: 49g; Fiber: 9g; Protein: 12g

MAKE-AHEAD TIP: You can make several servings ahead of time so you have them ready to go for the week. You can also substitute other fruit, add nuts, etc. Get creative!

HEALING CHICKEN GINGER SOUP

NAUSEA FIGHTER, VEGGIE LOADED

SERVES 8 / PREP TIME: 30 MINUTES / COOK TIME: 1 HOUR 30 MINUTES

The first trimester often includes nausea, a loss of appetite, and powerful food cravings. What better way to get in some quality nutrients and help reduce the nausea than with some chicken soup? This recipe includes ginger to help settle nausea and a variety of nutritious ingredients that support the health of you and your baby.

2 tablespoons extra-virgin olive oil

1 medium onion, chopped

3 garlic cloves, minced

2 medium carrots, chopped

2 medium celery stalks, chopped

1 tablespoon peeled minced fresh ginger

2 teaspoons dried parsley

½ teaspoon black pepper

8 cups chicken broth

1 bay leaf

1½ pounds chicken breasts, chopped

2 teaspoons Adobo seasoning

¼ cup rolled oats

2 cups chopped kale

1. In a stock pot, heat the olive oil on medium heat until shimmering, about 3 minutes.
2. Add the onion and cook until translucent, about 2 minutes.
3. Add garlic, carrots, celery, ginger, parsley, and pepper. Let cook for 4 to 5 minutes, stirring occasionally.
4. Add the chicken broth and bay leaf. Turn the heat to high.
5. Season the chicken with Adobo.
6. Once the broth begins to boil, add the chicken. Turn the heat to low and let the chicken cook through, about 5 minutes.
7. Add the oats, cover the pot, and simmer for 1 hour.
8. Add the kale and let cook uncovered until wilted, about 2 minutes. Serve.

PER SERVING: Calories: 160; Total fat: 6g; Saturated fat: 1g; Cholesterol: 60mg; Sodium: 851mg; Carbohydrates: 6g; Fiber: 1g; Protein: 21g

PREP TIP: You can add salt to taste, but you may not need to with the Adobo seasoning. Omit the oats for a thinner, lighter soup.

SALMON VEGGIE BOWL

PROTEIN POWER, VEGGIE LOADED / SERVES 2 / PREP TIME: 30 MINUTES, PLUS 3 HOURS TO MARINATE / COOK TIME: 10 MINUTES

Many women prefer cold foods during the first trimester, so this bowl is a perfect meal to nourish you and your baby. Salmon contains healthy fats and low levels of mercury. The leafy greens in the recipe provide important nutrients, such as folate, which is important for the development of a baby's central nervous system.

FOR THE MARINADE

Juice of 1 lemon or
2 tablespoons bottled
lemon juice

2 teaspoons honey

1 garlic clove, minced

2 tablespoons extra-virgin
olive oil

FOR THE BOWL

1 cup chopped romaine
lettuce

1 medium tomato,
chopped

1 cup pinto beans, drained
(precooked or canned)

1 medium carrot,
shredded

½ cup chopped cilantro

¼ red onion, chopped

1 cup cooked rice

2 4-ounce salmon fillets

1 tablespoon extra-virgin
olive oil

½ avocado, sliced

TO MAKE THE MARINADE

1. In a small bowl, mix together the lemon juice, honey, garlic, and olive oil.
2. Put the salmon in a resealable plastic bag or bowl, cover with the marinade, and refrigerate for at least 3 hours.

TO MAKE THE BOWL

3. Divide the lettuce, tomato, beans, carrot, cilantro, onion, and rice between two large salad bowls.
4. Heat a sauté pan over medium-high heat. Add the olive oil. Add the salmon and cook 3 to 4 minutes on each side or until cooked through.
5. Add half the salmon to each bowl and top with the sliced avocado.

continued on next page ⋯→

continued from previous page

FOR THE DRESSING

2 teaspoons honey

2 tablespoons extra-virgin olive oil

Juice of 1 lemon or 2 tablespoons lemon juice

¼ teaspoon garlic powder

⅛ teaspoon black pepper

¼ teaspoon sea salt

TO MAKE THE DRESSING

6. While the salmon is cooking, whisk the honey, olive oil, lemon juice, garlic powder, pepper, and salt in a separate, small bowl.

7. Top each bowl with half of the dressing. Toss and serve.

PER SERVING: Calories: 732; Total fat: 38g; Saturated fat: 6g; Cholesterol: 55mg; Sodium: 497mg; Carbohydrates: 68g; Fiber: 13g; Protein: 34g

SUBSTITUTION TIP: You can make substitutions based on your taste preferences, using different types of fish, black beans instead of pinto beans, or spinach instead of romaine lettuce.

FIGHT THE NAUSEA SMOOTHIE

LIGHT BITE, NAUSEA FIGHTER

SERVES 2 / PREP TIME: 5 MINUTES

This smoothie is simple to make and is a wonderful remedy for first-trimester nausea. It is easy on the stomach and provides excellent nourishment from a variety of vegetables and fruits. Spinach is a great source of folate, an important nutrient during your first trimester.

1 tablespoon peeled sliced fresh ginger

1 cup frozen pineapple

½ medium cucumber, peeled and chopped

½ cup fresh spinach

1 banana

Juice of ½ lemon or 1 tablespoon bottled lemon juice

1 cup water

Put the ginger, pineapple, cucumber, spinach, banana, lemon juice, and water in a blender and blend well. Serve immediately.

PER SERVING: Calories: 104; Total fat: <1g; Saturated fat: <1g; Cholesterol: 0mg; Sodium: 8mg; Carbohydrates: 26g; Fiber: 3g; Protein: 2g

PREP TIP: You can use canned pineapple in its natural juices. You can also use other leafy greens that are high in folate, such as kale, instead of spinach.

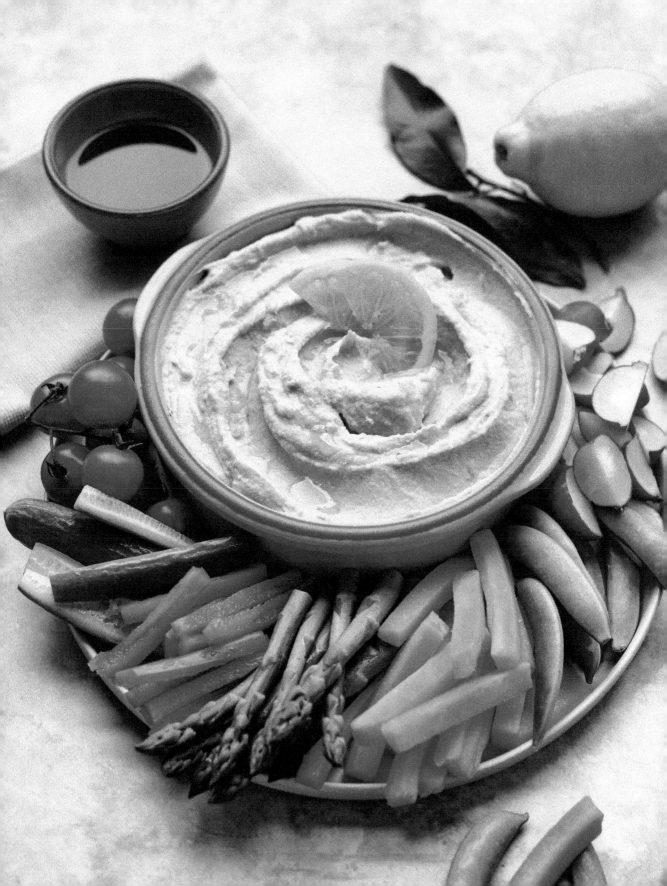

LEMON GARLIC HUMMUS

PROTEIN POWER, QUICK AND EASY

SERVES 10 / PREP TIME: 10 MINUTES

Hummus is a great way to make raw vegetables more appetizing. This recipe contains healthy fats from the olive oil, tahini (ground sesame seeds), and chickpeas. It's a great first-trimester food because it delivers simple flavors that are easy to digest.

2 cups cooked or canned chickpeas

Juice of 2 lemons or 4 tablespoons bottled lemon juice

¾ teaspoon sea salt

3 garlic cloves, minced

2 teaspoons tahini

2 teaspoons extra-virgin olive oil

1. Combine the chickpeas, lemon juice, salt, garlic, tahini, and olive oil in a blender or food processor. Blend until smooth.
2. To serve, pair with vegetables of choice for dipping: carrot or celery sticks, bell pepper slices, cherry tomatoes, cucumber, radishes, sugar snap peas, etc.

PER SERVING: Calories: 71; Total fat: 2g; Saturated fat: <1g; Cholesterol: 0mg; Sodium: 179mg; Carbohydrates: 10g; Fiber: 3g; Protein: 3g

PREP TIP: You can cook the chickpeas in a digital pressure cooker. If you want the hummus thinner, add more lemon juice and/or olive oil to get the desired consistency. Adding a small amount of cold water can also help make the hummus smoother.

TO CBD OR NOT TO CBD?

Pregnancy and breastfeeding may be two of the most emotionally and physically intense life experiences you'll ever have. Using cannabidiol (CBD) to deal with pain and other common pregnancy-related ailments, such as nausea, insomnia, depression, and/or anxiety, is a growing trend among women looking for an alternative to modern pharmaceutical drugs. Unlike tetrahydrocannabinol (THC), marijuana's most active ingredient that is responsible for the "high" feeling, CBD is indeed medicinal. However, since there is insufficient research on the use of CBD oil during pregnancy, most experts, practitioners, the FDA, and women's health governing bodies suggest avoiding it.

Similar to other medications and drugs, some chemicals ingested during marijuana use can pass through the placenta and through breast milk, *potentially* affecting healthy fetal brain development and increasing your risk of giving birth to a preterm, low–birth weight, or stillborn baby. If you want to try CBD oil during pregnancy, talk to your provider and have a candid conversation about your intentions so that everyone involved is on the same page. There are a range of options to help you manage the unpleasant symptoms associated with pregnancy and postpartum. If you have the urge to try CBD oil, it's best to do it *before* or *after* your pregnancy and postpartum periods so that you know how your body will respond.

Essential Oil Blends for the First Trimester

This section contains essential oil blends designed to alleviate some common ailments you may encounter during the first trimester.

MORNING SICKNESS/NAUSEA

Ginger essential oil prevents vomiting and alleviates the intensity and frequency of queasiness. This essential oil works well for uncomfortable stomach issues like indigestion and bloating. You can diffuse up to 10 drops of Ginger essential oil as often as needed while alternating with other remedies. If necessary, you can rub diluted Ginger essential oil directly on your abdomen to improve nausea; however, the simplest way of using this oil is to slowly inhale it directly out of the bottle. *Note: Projectile vomiting or severe cases (hyperemesis gravidarum) may require hospital treatment due to the risk of liver disease and dehydration.

CONSTIPATION

Constipation, a symptom of other health problems, points directly to poor diet, sluggish digestion or muscle tone, and possibly nervous tension, which inhibits bowel movements. Rosemary essential oil revives the digestive system and stimulates bowel movement by improving gut circulation which boosts muscle contractions in the digestive tract for optimal digestion. Place three to five drops of Rosemary essential oil into your herbal tea before drinking.

Black Pepper essential oil is also helpful—it not only kick-starts the digestive system but also reduces inflammation. For best results, use two drops of Black Pepper essential oil instead of sprinkling ground black pepper on your food.

FATIGUE

Your body is working hard to create and support new life. Fatigue may very well be your biggest complaint during the first trimester of pregnancy. Although drinking coffee and other caffeinated beverages might sound like a convenient solution, these easy pick-me-ups put an extra burden on your already overworked adrenal glands and will actually worsen your fatigue. Instead, try massaging yourself with this blend: four drops of Pine essential oil, four drops of Spruce essential oil, two drops of Lavender essential oil, and one ounce of your preferred carrier oil. For extra invigoration, you can add two drops of Rosemary essential oil. And remember—schedule time to relax.

MOOD SWINGS (DEPRESSION/ANXIETY)

Emotionally, the first trimester can be difficult to manage. Your body is going through so many hormonal changes. Neroli essential oil addresses emotional instability and your inability to relax. To use, mix 20 drops of Neroli oil in four teaspoons of almond carrier oil and massage on the back of your neck, forehead, or temples. You can also blend with 5 to 10 drops of Lavender essential oil to enhance the effects. Ylang Ylang essential oil also doubles as a mood elevator and stress reliever by harmonizing and decreasing blood pressure, and helping you stay alert and attentive. Place 10 drops in your diffuser to uplift your mood.

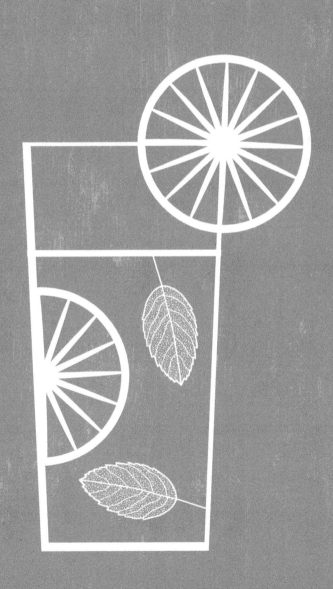

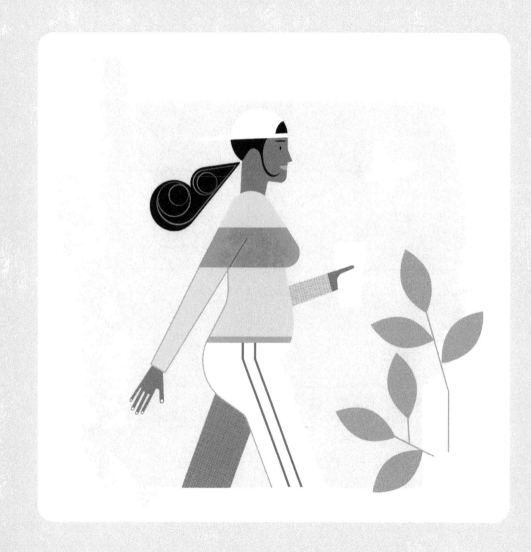

CHAPTER FIVE

The Second Trimester

One down, two to go! You and your baby have arrived at the second trimester, which, for many moms, is the best trimester of the three. Your early pregnancy symptoms are slowly yet progressively subsiding (notice how food is starting to smell and taste good for the first time in a while?). Despite your rising energy levels, you will still need your rest, but it won't feel like an all-day compulsion. You will also get a reprieve from going to the bathroom all day and night. Your breasts will keep getting bigger; however, they will not feel nearly as tender. By the end of week 17, you will begin to recognize changes in your lower abdomen as your baby bump starts to show. At some point in the middle of this trimester, you will feel your baby move for the first time. Fetal movement, called "quickening," can feel like twinges, flutters, bubbles, or even gas.

Even though you are only about halfway through your pregnancy, the experience is becoming more real by the moment. By the end of the second trimester, your baby will have grown considerably, and you (and others) will become acutely (and sometimes visibly) aware of daily fetal movements, which will feel more like kicks or punches. At the end of week 26, your pregnancy is more than halfway over, yet your baby has more growing to do. This can make the third trimester a lot more physically demanding, so take advantage of this time while you can still see your feet.

How's My Baby?

At the start of the second trimester, your baby is about four inches long (using standard "crown to rump" measurements), weighs about an ounce, and is the size of your fist. By the end of this trimester, your baby will measure a little more than nine inches and weigh about two pounds. To keep this growth going, you will need an extra 300 calories in your daily diet, which is absolutely necessary to support the development of your baby's cardio-vascular, nervous, integument (skin), and digestive systems. Eating smaller meals accompanied by several daily snacks is the perfect way to meet this requirement.

Food cravings and aversions will be more prevalent during this time in your pregnancy. Even if you are craving sweets, it is important to avoid artificial sweeteners like saccharin and aspartame, as these additives are harmful to your baby. The amniotic fluid that surrounds your baby is flavored by the foods you eat, so your baby is getting a daily sampling of your meals. For this reason, it's important to keep track of your sodium intake because excess sodium will lead to unnecessary swelling and bloating. During the course of this trimester, your baby will start looking more like the newborn you will see in about three months. Your baby can now perceive light and darkness, voices, your heartbeat and stomach gurgles, dog barking, sirens, and loud television. Toward the end of the second trimester their eyes begin to open. You may even be able to feel their hiccups.

How Am I?

Investing in maternity clothes is a sound decision right now. Don't manage your growing abdomen by not buttoning or zipping your pants all the way or employing safety pins to extend your waistband. You will enjoy your pregnancy more with clothing that fits comfortably. Emotionally, you may be feeling scattered and unfocused. You may also be feeling excitement, and possibly some misgivings, about "showing."

Now that your early pregnancy symptoms have subsided, you will have more energy and may have more interest in having sex. You may be more likely to have multiple orgasms due to the extra blood flow to the labia, clitoris, and vagina. At the midpoint of your pregnancy, 20 weeks, your uterus measures at the level of your navel so you will need to begin sleeping on your left side. Putting some pillows behind you when you sleep will prevent you from rolling over so you will not lie flat on your back. By the end of the second trimester, your uterus will be about two and a half inches above your belly button and you will have healthily gained about 19 pounds.

How's My Pregnancy?

In your second trimester, your practitioner will check on your weight, blood pressure, and fetal heartbeat. A quad screen, while not conducted on all pregnant women, measures alpha-fetoprotein, hCG, unconjugated estradiol, and inhibin-A levels in order to determine the presence of Down syndrome. Your practitioner will also conduct a urinalysis and manually evaluate the size of your uterus.

You may have several practical concerns about your pregnancy ranging from how your behavior affects your baby's development to the changing dynamics between you and your partner. Keep a list of the questions, symptoms, and challenges you are experiencing so you can discuss them at each appointment. If you are nervous, or unsure if something is important or serious during your pregnancy, just ask. Don't be embarrassed! It's better to ask questions, even if only for your own peace of mind. A good provider will take the best possible care of you and your baby. He or she will honor any preferences you have, as long as they are reasonable and workable. That said, get ready to be flexible. There will be much about your pregnancy and birth that you can't predict, but preparing in a healthy way and advocating for what you do want will go a long way toward keeping your pregnancy and delivery smooth and setting your mind at ease.

Even though you are taking a prenatal vitamin, you may still develop iron deficiency anemia during pregnancy as your baby uses some of the iron stored in your body. Iron is the most important supplement to take during pregnancy, so be sure to take a prenatal vitamin that contains iron.

Sign up for childbirth classes if possible, practice your childbirth preparation exercises, and become familiar with the birth process. This is also the perfect time to think about hiring a doula to be your labor support specialist. Your doula can help you plan an advanced tour of the facility where you will deliver your baby and also help you choose the appropriate childbirth education classes. Your doula can help you devise your birth plan and help you carry it out. Besides learning childbirth techniques, sign up for an infant CPR and first-aid class. There is no time like the present to keep your newborn safe and sound.

The Aches and Pains

Growing a baby inside you is a lot of work, and rarely comfortable. You expect that labor and delivery will be painful, but what is happening to you right now? Your body is changing in many ways and in many directions, all at the same time. As your baby grows and develops, your uterus does, too. This means back, abdomen, groin, and thigh aches and pains accompany all the other "joys" of pregnancy. As your baby grows, the pressure of its head, your increased weight, and the loosening of your joints can contribute to backaches and pain near your pelvic bone. If the uterus pinches the sciatic nerve you may experience shooting pain that runs from the lower back down the back of one leg. If this is your first pregnancy, your baby's growth and the resulting discomfort may be surprising. Sometimes the pain will be agonizing; however, safe options for pain relief are available. Here are some treatments for the common aches and pains of the second trimester.

HEARTBURN

Heartburn, that burning feeling in your throat and chest, is a symptom of indigestion. It happens as hormones relax the smooth muscle tissue in your gastrointestinal tract. While uncomfortable for you, heartburn actually benefits your baby. Slower digestion improves the absorption of nutrients into your bloodstream through the placenta and on to your baby. In addition, the hormones responsible for your frequent heartburn, relaxin and progesterone, also cause fetal hair growth, so it's likely that if you're having a lot of heartburn your baby will be born with a full head of hair. Instead of eating three large meals, opt for five or six smaller, balanced, nutritious ones to feel better. In addition, any food that triggers heartburn should be taken off the menu for now. Spicy foods, fried foods, fatty foods, highly seasoned foods, chocolate, mint, coffee, carbonated beverages, and processed meats are likely offenders. Also, keep some sugarless chewing gum in your purse or handbag and try using it about 30 minutes after eating. The act of chewing reduces excess acid by triggering a digestive response.

ROUND LIGAMENT PAIN

Equivalent to "growing pains," round ligament pain is the result of the stretching of muscles and ligaments that support your growing uterus. It may show up as unilateral sharp, stabbing cramps or dull abdominal aches upon rising from a seated position or when you cough. To relieve and prevent these pains, try to avoid abrupt changes in position. When you move, turn your entire body rather than just turning at your waist. Bending toward the pain will also help relieve the sensation. Even though this symptom is physiologically common, mention it to your provider at your next visit.

STRETCH MARKS

During pregnancy, stretch marks may appear on your breasts, abdomen, hips, and buttocks. Gaining weight gradually is the best way to help minimize the marks. You can also promote skin elasticity with a balanced diet rich in vitamin C. After pregnancy, the marks will fade, but they will not disappear; however, there is no harm in applying moisturizers. Avoid steroid creams, as you will absorb them into your bloodstream and they can pass on to your developing baby. There are no miracle creams that prevent stretch marks. The only treatments for stretch marks, laser therapy and prescriptions containing glycolic acid, can be implemented *after* pregnancy.

LEG CRAMPS

Nighttime calf cramps can disrupt your much-needed sleep. Before going to bed, try stretching your legs first. If cramps still wake you up, massage your calf with long, downward strokes. Straighten your leg and slowly flex your entire foot toward your nose. When possible, avoid standing for long periods and wear compression stockings during the day. You can also use a heating pad on the affected calf, but do not use it for longer than 15 minutes at a time. For severe and persistent cramps, contact your practitioner to rule out the emergent possibility of blood clot formation.

DENTAL ISSUES

Pregnant women are at increased risk for cavities and gum disease. Your gums may swell and bleed due to pregnancy hormones, but continue brushing and flossing as usual. Mouthwash and gargles are fine to use. Switching to a softer toothbrush may help your gums feel less irritated. If you have a dentist appointment already scheduled, keep it. A dental checkup in pregnancy ensures that your mouth is healthy. If you need local anesthesia or dental x-rays, let your dentist know that you are pregnant so they can protect your thyroid with a shield. As always, consult your provider before taking any medications.

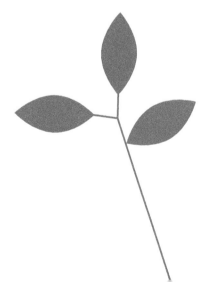

The Best Exercises

Exercise not only affects *your* health, but also the health of your developing baby. For low-risk pregnancies, exercise or be active for a total of 30 minutes each day. Working out while pregnant also gives you a head start in getting your body back after delivery. A light exercise and stretching routine in the second trimester can help alleviate a host of conditions and assist in proper fetal positioning, which makes birth easier. If your pregnancy is high risk or if you have had several miscarriages, discuss exercise with your provider before starting an activity. Listen to your body; it will tell you when it is time to slow down. Due to your growing uterus, your body is heavier, and this will ultimately affect your sense of balance. Keep these changes in mind as you adjust your workouts. Here are some suggestions for healthy ways to keep active in your second trimester.

WALKING

There is no easier exercise to fit into your schedule than walking. There is also no special equipment necessary (except supportive, comfortable shoes), and you do not need to pay for gym memberships. The best part? All the walking you do throughout the course of your day counts! Whether it is walking to the farmers' market, parking farther away at the store, or the 10 minutes you spend walking the dog, use these situations to your advantage.

The good news is that you can continue walking right up to delivery, and walking will help aid the natural progression of your contractions. If you weren't active before getting pregnant, walking is as involved as you should get with exercise (swimming is also low impact enough to take on). Walking briskly for 30 minutes every day is the quintessential way to incorporate exercise into your lifestyle. Begin slowly with casual strolling before progressing to a brisk pace. Walking alone gives you the opportunity to quiet your mind, and you can also enjoy the additional benefits of forest bathing. If you would rather have company, invite your partner, friends, or colleagues. You can even join a Meetup group for pregnant women. If the weather doesn't cooperate, you can always join the mall walkers.

STRETCHES

Stretching is a great way to stay healthy and ward off some nasty aches and pains. Try the following routines to see which work best for you.

HIP FLEXORS

1. Face the stairs, using the wall or railing for support.

2. Put one foot on a step and bend your knee while keeping the other leg straight.

3. Lean into your bent leg, keeping your back straight.

4. Feel the stretch in your straight leg.

5. Switch legs and repeat on the other side.

PSOAS STRETCH

1. Lie on your back, using pillows to create a diagonal from your lower back to your head.

2. Bend your knees with your heels a foot away from your buttocks, about hip-width apart.

3. With your hands at your sides, rest in this position for 15 minutes.

FORWARD-LEANING INVERSION

1. Kneel on the edge of the bed.

2. Lower yourself to the floor, resting on your forearms.

3. Let your head hang freely, chin tucked.

4. Slowly sway your hips.

5. Flatten your lower back.

6. Take three deep breaths.

7. Return to the kneeling position.

1. Stand with your feet shoulder-width apart.

2. With your back straight, slowly lower yourself as close to the ground as possible. If this is challenging, move your feet farther apart.

3. Hold the squat for 30 seconds.

4. Slowly come back to a standing position.

5. Repeat five times.

LABOR LUNGES

During the second trimester, avoid "walking" lunges (forward lunges) as relaxed joints are more prone to injury. However, "labor" lunges are a good exercise to help open your pelvis during labor and delivery if you are planning for a vaginal birth. To do labor lunges, open one leg and lunge out to the side of your body. Propping up your foot on a stool or low chair will help your baby move down lower into your pelvis, a better position for birth. During contractions, you can lunge from one side to the other between contractions.

MATERNAL POSITIONING

Improper seated positions put undue stress on your spine. At home, practice sitting erect, accentuating the curve of your back, with your shoulders rounded backward and your buttocks touching the back of your chair. Hold this position for a few seconds and then *slightly* relax. To keep your hips at a 90-degree angle, use a footrest to elevate your feet. Use chairs that provide good support with a straight back, arms, and a cushion. For extra support, place a rolled-up towel or a lumbar roll in the hollow of your back. Prolonged sitting may also prove to be troublesome for your back, so avoid sitting in the same position for more than 30 minutes. At work, trade your office chair for a maternity or exercise ball. The maternity ball will comfort and strengthen your lower back while keeping your pelvis open and supported. To be fair, you may not be able to sit comfortably upright without a few practice attempts. To sit properly using the maternity ball, sit so that your feet and the center of the ball make a tripod. A properly inflated ball will be big enough so that your hips are equal to or higher than your knees.

Sex and the Babymoon

During the second trimester your libido will make a brief yet intense return after a tumultuous first trimester. Your body will start to feel somewhat normal and your hormone surge can have a variety of effects on arousal, pleasure, desire, and intimacy. A *babymoon* is an opportunity for expectant mothers and their partners to vacation alone as a couple before the baby arrives, reality sets in, and the transition from couple to family begins.

When considering where to go, think about places and locations where you and your partner can spend time relaxing and enjoying each other before the sleepless nights start. Whether you vacation to a beautiful beach, enjoy a long weekend at a spa, or have an extended stay at a luxury hotel, the main themes are relaxation, partnership, and fun. This time in your pregnancy is an opportunity for rekindling closeness and intimacy, and sex can be a positive part of this experience. If your pregnancy is low risk and uncomplicated, sex (and orgasms) will not hurt your baby. The amniotic sac protects against germs and seminal fluid. As your baby grows, sexual intercourse may become difficult because you are physically uncomfortable. Changing positions (side-lying, being on top, and entry from behind) will enable you to continue enjoying sex during this part of your pregnancy. If you and your partner have concerns about sex during pregnancy, discuss them openly and bring them to your provider together.

GESTATIONAL DIABETES

If you have not had diabetes before but you develop it during pregnancy, it is called *gestational diabetes* (GD). During pregnancy, if you produce less insulin or if your body cannot use insulin appropriately, your blood sugar levels will be high. GD develops between weeks 24 and 28, which is why your provider schedules a routine glucose screening test at 28 weeks. You probably won't show any symptoms even if you do develop GD, but you may experience unusual thirst, overabundant urination, and fatigue. Sugar will be detectable in the urine. A glucose tolerance test follows a glucose screening test if the screening test shows high glucose levels. The tolerance test, done while fasting and on an empty stomach, lasts longer, about three hours, and requires four blood samples.

Untreated, GD has serious repercussions for you and your baby, as you both will be exposed to an unhealthy concentration of sugar. You might have excessive amounts of amniotic fluid, which will swell your uterus and can cause premature labor. You may also have a long labor because your baby is large and cannot fit through the birth canal. In this instance, a cesarean delivery will be required. With high blood sugar, you may experience frequent infections of the kidneys, bladder, cervix, and uterus. You can prevent and treat GD by maintaining a healthy weight, both before and during pregnancy, eating a healthy diet, avoiding refined sugar, exercising regularly, and getting enough folic acid from a balanced diet, 0.8 to 1 milligram a day.

Recipes for the Second Trimester

LOADED VEGGIE BREAKFAST CASSEROLE

PROTEIN POWER, VEGGIE LOADED

SERVES 12 / PREP TIME: 15 MINUTES / COOK TIME: 1 HOUR

By now you should be feeling a little better than during the first trimester and ready to try out some new, healthy recipes. This recipe provides some nutrition basics for healthy eating during pregnancy: protein, healthy fats, and plenty of vegetables. Eggs are an excellent source of protein and healthy fat for mom and her developing baby.

1 tablespoon extra-virgin olive oil

1 sweet onion, chopped

1 head of broccoli, chopped

8 ounces mushrooms, sliced

1 teaspoon garlic powder

1 teaspoon dried parsley

1 teaspoon sea salt

½ teaspoon black pepper

10 large eggs

½ cup unsweetened almond milk

8 ounces shredded cheddar

1 pint grape tomatoes, halved

1. Preheat the oven to 350°F.
2. Heat the olive oil in a sauté pan on medium-high heat.
3. Add the onion, broccoli, mushrooms, garlic powder, parsley, salt, and pepper. Sauté until cooked through, about 5 minutes.
4. Spread the cooked vegetables across the bottom of a 9-by-14-inch greased baking dish.
5. Whisk the eggs and almond milk together, then pour the egg mixture on top of the cooked vegetables.
6. Top with cheese, then the grape tomato halves.
7. Bake for 50 minutes or until eggs set and the top starts to turn a golden brown. Serve.

PER SERVING: Calories: 174; Total fat: 12g; Saturated fat: 5g; Cholesterol: 154mg; Sodium: 389mg; Carbohydrates: 7g; Fiber: 2g; Protein: 12g

MAKE-AHEAD TIP: If you are pressed for time in the mornings, prepare the vegetables the night before.

BALSAMIC CHICKEN LENTIL SALAD

**PROTEIN POWER / SERVES 6 / PREP TIME: 20 MINUTES,
PLUS 3 HOURS TO MARINATE / COOK TIME: 30 MINUTES**

*Additional protein is often encouraged for pregnant women. This salad
includes excellent protein sources mixed with nourishing veggies.*

FOR THE MARINADE

2 tablespoons extra-virgin
olive oil

3 tablespoons balsamic
vinegar

2 garlic cloves, minced

¼ teaspoon sea salt

½ teaspoon black pepper

½ teaspoon dried
rosemary

1½ pounds chicken, cut
into strips

FOR THE SALAD

3 cups cooked lentils

¼ teaspoon garlic powder

1 teaspoon sea salt

½ teaspoon black pepper

2 tablespoons extra-virgin
olive oil, divided

2 tomatoes, chopped

1 cucumber, diced

1 cup chopped fresh
cilantro

5 scallions, chopped

Juice of ½ lemon or
1 tablespoon bottled
lemon juice

TO MAKE THE MARINADE

1. In a medium bowl or resealable plastic bag,
   combine the olive oil, vinegar, garlic, salt, pepper,
   and rosemary, mixing well.
2. Add the chicken strips, tossing to coat well, and
   marinate for at least 3 hours.

TO MAKE THE SALAD

3. Toss the lentils, garlic powder, salt, and pepper
   together and set aside.
4. Heat a medium skillet over medium-high heat.
   Add 1 tablespoon oil and heat until oil is hot and
   shimmering, about 1 minute.
5. Add the chicken. Cook until the meat is no longer
   pink and heated through, about 4 minutes on
   each side.
6. While the chicken cooks, toss the tomatoes,
   cucumber, cilantro, and scallions together, then
   drizzle with 1 tablespoon oil and the lemon juice.
7. Top with the chicken and lentils and serve.

PER SERVING: Calories: 328; Total fat: 10g; Saturated fat: 2g;
Cholesterol: 80mg; Sodium: 498mg; Carbohydrates: 25g; Fiber: 7g;
Protein: 35g

PREP TIP: If using dry lentils, soak them in a bowl
of water overnight. Then strain, put in a pot, and
cover with water. Bring them to a boil, then simmer
until the lentils are plump and tender, about
15 minutes. Drain and cool to room temperature.

ONE LAYER EGGPLANT LASAGNA

VEGGIE LOADED

SERVES 6 / PREP TIME: 15 MINUTES / COOK TIME: 1 HOUR

Healthy eating does not have to be complicated! This dish is simple yet nutritious, a noodle-free lasagna that won't weigh you down with too many starches. Instead you will get protein, healthy fats, and vegetables to meet a variety of nutrient needs during trimester two.

1 tablespoon extra-virgin olive oil

1 pound ground beef (preferably grass-fed)

1 tablespoon Italian seasoning

1 (16-ounce) jar organic tomato sauce

1 medium eggplant, cut into 1-inch rounds (not peeled)

2 cups fresh spinach

8 ounces shredded mozzarella (or shredded vegan mozzarella)

1. Preheat the oven to 375°F.
2. Heat the olive oil in a sauté pan on medium-high heat. Add the ground beef and Italian seasoning and cook until the meat is no longer pink, stirring often.
3. Spread 3 tablespoons of the tomato sauce around the bottom of a 9-by-13-inch casserole dish. Line with the eggplant slices.
4. Layer with the cooked ground beef, then spinach, then sauce. Top with mozzarella cheese.
5. Bake for 45 minutes. Let rest for 10 minutes and serve.

PER SERVING: Calories: 336; Total fat: 20g; Saturated fat: 9g; Cholesterol: 71mg; Sodium: 697mg; Carbohydrates: 15g; Fiber: 5g; Protein: 26g

SUBSTITUTION TIP: Feel free to add mushrooms or other vegetables you like. Vegan mozzarella can also work well in this recipe; many vegan varieties taste best when melted.

NOURISHING TROPICAL SMOOTHIE

LIGHT BITE, QUICK AND EASY

SERVES 1 / PREP TIME: 5 MINUTES

Smoothies are a great option for a treat that's convenient and nourishing. You can load them up with fruits and vegetables to get in a good amount of fiber and a variety of nutrients like folate and vitamin C. The collagen peptides in this recipe are an excellent protein source, which is important to meet the needs of your growing baby.

1 cup frozen tropical
fruit mix

1½ cups unsweetened
almond milk

1 tablespoon coconut oil

2 tablespoons collagen
peptides

½ cup fresh spinach

1 small mandarin orange,
peeled and seeded

Combine the fruit mix, almond milk, coconut oil, collagen peptides, spinach, and orange in a blender and blend well. Serve immediately.

PER SERVING: Calories: 349; Total fat: 18g; Saturated fat: 11g; Cholesterol: 0mg; Sodium: 269mg; Carbohydrates: 36g; Fiber: 5g; Protein: 14g

PREP TIP: Collagen peptides are quite popular and can be found at most stores or online. Aim for good quality ones from grass-fed, pasture-raised animals. If you can't find them, use unflavored gelatin or a good quality protein powder.

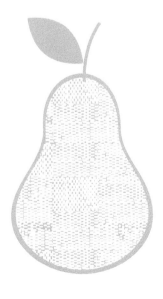

CARROT AND ZUCCHINI MAPLE MUFFINS

**VEGGIE LOADED / MAKES 20 MUFFINS / PREP TIME: 15 MINUTES
COOK TIME: 20 MINUTES**

We all want a sweet treat from time to time. This recipe will satisfy your sweet tooth with vegetables instead of processed sugar. You can feel good about snacking on it!

¾ cup coconut flour

1 teaspoon baking soda

½ teaspoon sea salt

½ teaspoon cinnamon

3 large eggs

1 tablespoon unsweetened almond milk

⅓ cup maple syrup

1 teaspoon vanilla extract

⅔ cup unsweetened applesauce

⅓ cup coconut oil, melted

1 cup shredded zucchini

½ cup shredded carrot

1. Preheat the oven to 350°F. Grease a muffin pan or line with muffin liners.
2. In a bowl, mix together the coconut flour, baking soda, salt, and cinnamon.
3. In a separate bowl, whisk together the eggs and the almond milk.
4. In a third bowl, combine the maple syrup, vanilla extract, applesauce, and melted coconut oil.
5. Add the egg mixture to the dry ingredient mixture. Stir to combine.
6. Add the applesauce mixture and stir to combine.
7. Fold in the zucchini and carrot.
8. Evenly distribute the batter into the prepared muffin pan, filling each section ¾ full.
9. Bake for 20 minutes. Cool for 10 minutes and serve.

PER SERVING (1 muffin): Calories: 81; Total fat: 5g; Saturated fat: 4g; Cholesterol: 25mg; Sodium: 142mg; Carbohydrates: 7g; Fiber: 2g; Protein: 2g

MAKE-AHEAD TIP: These are great as a snack, as a dessert, or for a quick breakfast. They make a great healthy and easy snack during the postpartum period as well. Make a big batch and freeze it, reheating for 30 seconds in the microwave.

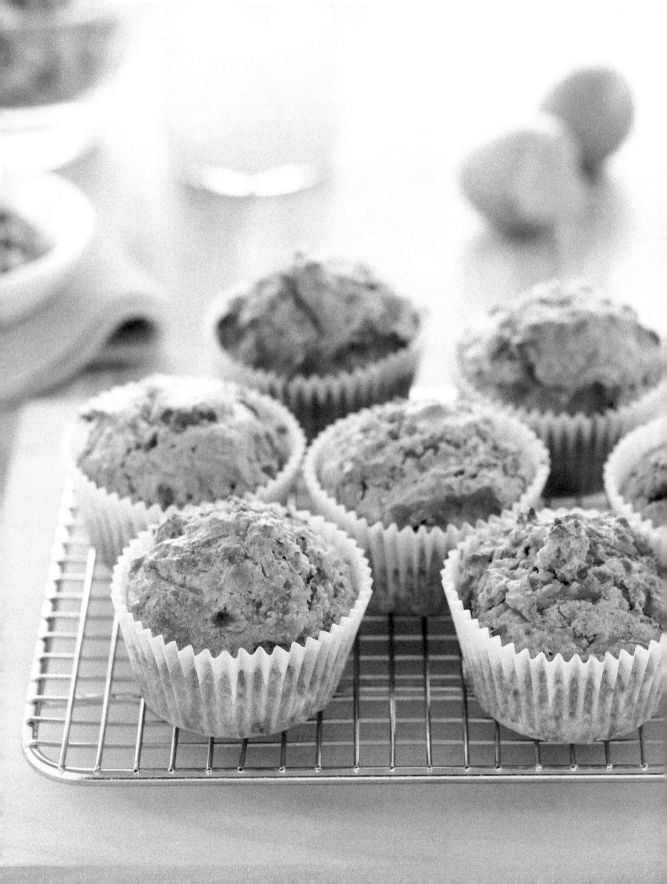

Essential Oil Blends for the Second Trimester

This section contains essential oil blends designed to alleviate some common ailments you may encounter during the second trimester.

HEARTBURN

The easiest way to treat heartburn with essential oils is by inhaling the peppermint scent directly from the bottle. Should you choose to use a diffuser, add two or three drops to the water. If time is of the essence, you can also breathe deeply while hovering over a cloth napkin or washcloth infused with three drops of Peppermint essential oil. For more immediate relief, take a shot of almond milk with two drops of Peppermint oil added. Another option, if tolerable, is to add three drops of Peppermint essential oil to 8 ounces of water and sip throughout the day.

LEG CRAMPS

To soothe active leg cramps or muscle spasms, use warm, moist heat with beneficial essential oils. Using one drop of Lavender oil and one drop of either Geranium, Grapefruit, Roman Chamomile, or White Fir essential oil, add two drops to a palmful of almond carrier oil. Massage over the entire cramping muscle for immediate relief. Another alternative is adding one drop of pain-relieving Lavender essential oil or spasm-reducing Chamomile essential oil (or two drops of a single oil) to one teaspoon of grapeseed oil, and massage away.

DENTAL ISSUES

Dental health is important all the way through your pregnancy. For an extra bacteria-fighting boost, try oil pulling, the process of swishing about one tablespoon of oil around in your mouth for about 20 minutes (yes, minutes) before spitting it out. For an even stronger boost, add two drops of essential oil to coconut oil before rinsing your mouth. You can also create a natural mouthwash by adding two essential oil drops to about an ounce of water prior to rinsing your mouth, or a drop of essential oil to a pea-size amount of toothpaste before brushing. To kill harmful bacteria that cause bad breath, use Peppermint, Tea Tree, Myrrh, or Eucalyptus essential oil. Tea Tree and Cinnamon essential oils are great for gingivitis because of their antimicrobial properties. Clove essential oil also treats gum disease and can relieve toothache. Rosemary, Clove, and Tea Tree essential oils help prevent cavities.

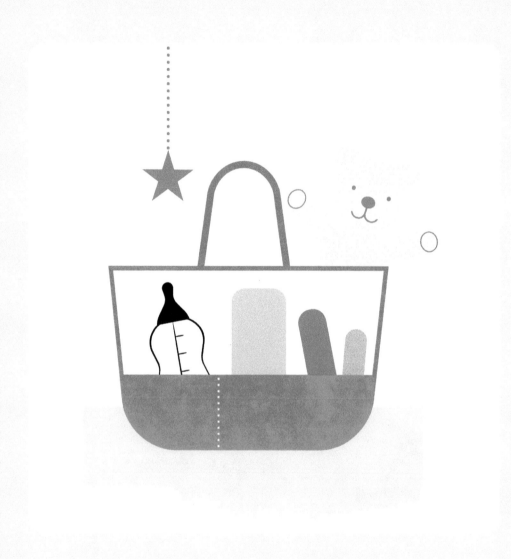

CHAPTER SIX

The Third Trimester

Welcome to your third trimester! You've passed the halfway mark and are about three months from delivery day. As the anticipation builds, you'll notice some of those annoying symptoms from the first trimester returning, and some new ones will also make an appearance. Since the main event is on the horizon, now is the time to commit to your childbirth education classes and/or hire a doula, if you haven't already. At this stage, you will be balancing the excitement of meeting your baby for the first time with the overall weariness of being pregnant. Don't worry—you've got this!

If this is your first baby, you might feel anxious about the unknowns. Reaching out to trusted friends and family for encouragement (not advice) will help you talk through your emotions while also establishing a village of support. During these last three months, you might feel woefully unprepared emotionally, physically, and mentally, even after spending the last six months doing exactly that—preparing. Even though you may be ready for pregnancy to be over so you can feel your baby in your arms (and see your feet again), you may feel like there is still so much to accomplish. The additional appointments, last-minute shopping, and preparation for maternity leave may leave you utterly exhausted. The tendency may be to focus on your due date as the end of the line, but try to carve out some time to create a welcoming postpartum space for you, your new-born, and your growing family. This chapter will help guide you through those decisions (and all the waiting) and offer insights on how to have a healthy, happy final trimester.

How's My Baby?

At the beginning of the third trimester, your baby weighs a little more than two pounds, measures about 16 inches, and is blinking. By the time your baby is born, it will weigh around 7.5 pounds and will be about 21.5 inches long, with little room for movement in your uterus. Be mindful of the fact that birth weight typically increases with each pregnancy.

Your baby's pokes and kicks are noticeably more uncomfortable now, as there is less amniotic fluid to absorb the shock. Despite that, feeling your baby move is still one of the most precious parts of pregnancy. Your baby's movements are reassuring—they're supposed to be wiggly!—and are an experience that both partners can enjoy. By week 37, your baby's head is usu-ally directed down into the pelvis. Week 38 is the milestone for a full-term infant. Fetal monitoring during labor enables your provider to detect any challenges early so that they can be resolved early. If you are still pregnant after week 38, your baby is still growing and gaining weight, just not as rapidly as before; however, all its organ systems are completely developed, including the lungs, which are the last organ to mature, and are where they need to be. As you near week 40 and your estimated due date, remember that you are not "overdue," or *postdates*, until 42 weeks of pregnancy.

How Am I?

At the beginning of the third trimester your uterus is about 12 inches from the top of your pubic bone. Even though you may feel like there's no more room in your womb for growth, believe it or not, you have more expanding to do. Physically, you are likely feeling stronger and feeling the baby move more frequently. You may have mild swelling of your ankles and feet, and occasionally your hands and face. Sitting with the right posture helps your circulation, so avoid crossing your legs (both at the knee and the ankle) to maintain adequate circulation. Swelling may also affect your hands and fingers, and you may notice that your rings or watches are tight. Your navel may start to stick out and those stretch marks become more noticeable. You may also begin to feel painless contractions as your uterus hardens momentarily. Although it seems early, your nipples may begin leaking colostrum, though this might not occur until after delivery.

Emotionally, you may feel incredibly excited . . . and also incredibly anxious as your due date approaches. You may notice strange and vivid dreams as well. Toward the end of your pregnancy, labor signs and symptoms will start to overshadow the other pregnancy symptoms that have developed along the way. Your weight gain slows as your due date approaches; however, lucky you—you have developed a distinct pregnancy waddle in preparation for the beginning of labor. You won't feel your baby moving as much, since they have less room to maneuver. Vaginal discharge becomes heavier, and you may notice streaks of red blood in your discharge after sex or after a pelvic exam. Remember all those trips to the bathroom during the first trimester? Well, they're back, as your baby increases in size and begins descending. Be prepared for alternating periods of tremendous fatigue and heightened energy (nesting syndrome).

How's My Pregnancy?

Midway through the third trimester, your provider will monitor your baby's growth and development through a nonstress test or a contraction stress test. This will further help confirm your baby's well-being while also detecting fetal challenges. You'll need to start thinking about post-birth logistics, like which approved car seat or child restraint system will work best for you as you take your baby home from the hospital. Even though delivery is still several weeks away, begin mapping out plans for your trip to the hospital. You will also want to choose a pediatrician for your newborn. Schedule a meeting in advance to get to know the provider and discuss your concerns and goals.

Together with your partner or doula, make a list of important numbers that will be needed before and after delivery. Always keep both lists with you, either written down or saved on your phone. Also, be mindful of your water breaking; it is not the large gush of water that is often portrayed on television, but rather a slow, continuous leak of clear fluid. As soon as your water breaks notify your provider. Your baby is getting ready to arrive!

Aches and Pains

It's been said before but it bears repeating: growing a human isn't easy. Just because your baby is almost here doesn't mean your pregnancy symptoms will slow down. You probably have so many different things running through your mind it may be hard to notice when pregnancy discomforts are intensifying, but you're not quite rid of them yet. In addition to fatigue, you may have increased swelling; remove your jewelry now while you still can. Restless legs, tingling, creeping, crawling sensations in your lower extremities, may also interfere with a sound night's sleep. To add insult to injury, you may have trouble breathing or feel winded with the slightest movement due to your growing uterus compressing your lungs. Thankfully, this feeling will subside once your baby begins to descend. You might also experience pressure under your ribs that will cause you some discomfort. If the pressure becomes pain, talk to your provider. Don't worry—all of the discomfort *will* pass. In the meantime, here are some tips to make your third-trimester aches and pains more bearable.

DRY SKIN

Hormonal changes strip your skin of oil, leaving you dry, scaly, and itchy. As always, the key to healthy skin is staying hydrated so keep drinking that water (see page 6). Omega-3 fats in the diet also complement properly hydrated skin. While staying hydrated, to keep your skin soft and supple, use a non-soap cleanser once a day, preferably something pH balanced and sulfate-free. In the shower, try wet skin moisturizers, an excellent addition to your skin care regimen. You can also slather yourself with an oil-based moisturizer (instead of a cream or lotion) after you bathe, while your skin is still damp. Use humidifiers in your rooms if dryness continues to be a nagging issue.

HEMORRHOIDS

Constipation can irritate and even cause hemorrhoids so hydration is key. Eating a high-fiber diet and incorporating dark leafy greens into each meal can also work wonders. Kegel exercises can stop the development of hemorrhoids by improving circulation to the perineum, the area between the vulva and the scrotum. Topical treatments, such as witch hazel and ice packs, soothe the skin and calm the discomfort of hemorrhoids. Warm baths coupled with doughnut-shaped pillows reduce discomfort by easing pressure in this area. Although it is a common treatment, avoid using mineral oil to combat hemorrhoids, as doing so will speed up the elimination of much-needed nutrients through the bowels.

VARICOSE VEINS

As pregnancy progresses, varicose veins become more noticeable and often increasingly more painful. Fortunately, in most cases, they do not cause a serious problem. However, you can help relieve the swelling and soreness. Once again, movement is key; light exercise such as walking or swimming helps maintain healthy circulation to your legs. Wearing support hose or compression stockings is also helpful if you find yourself standing for long periods of time during the day. When sitting, try not to cross your legs and use a footstool to prop up your feet.

REFLUX AND INDIGESTION

Here's that heartburn again. As mentioned earlier, heartburn and reflux are symptoms of indigestion. The last trimester does a number on your stomach as your uterus grows and presses against it. To put gastric juices and stomach acids in their rightful place, avoid eating while reclining or eating immediately before lying down. Stay away from foods and drinks that promote indigestion, like chocolate, coffee, carbonated drinks, spicy and highly seasoned foods, fried or fatty foods, processed meats and cheese, and mint. Also, less is more; enjoy six smaller meals throughout the day and eat slowly, taking small bites of food and intentionally chewing each bite.

BACK PAIN

An oversize abdomen and a pelvis weakened by loose joints often equals lower back pain. Luckily, there are several supports you can use to ease that discomfort. Invest in a support sling that relieves your back of the extra womb weight as your abdomen grows. Shoes with thicker, chunkier soles help align your body and keep you balanced and stable. Use an orthotic cushion in your shoes to provide additional support for your back. By the third trimester, you should not be lifting heavy loads above 20 pounds. Keep an eye on your posture as you sit to help prevent and ease discomfort in your lower back.

Last-Minute Preparations

Nesting—that urge to clean and organize to prepare your home for baby's arrival—is a real phenomenon. Take advantage of the extra energy, but ask for help when needed and accept assistance when it's offered. Get things in place so that they'll run more smoothly after the baby comes. Visit the grocery store and stock up on nutritious foods that can be prepared and served easily. Paper plates can be a lifesaver when the dishwasher is full. Take time to cook meals that are healthy and are also freezable, as these will be valuable when you are sleep-deprived. Remember that no matter what you plan, the baby can arrive unexpectedly, so stay flexible and prepare accordingly, as schedules and availability might get complicated. Take this time as an opportunity to involve your partner, family, and friends who are looking for meaningful ways to be helpful. Remember, you are human! You need to conserve your energy for the intense work of labor and delivery ahead.

BIRTH PLAN REVIEW

Your childbirth education classes provided you with guidance to prepare your birth plan, a written *idea* of what you would like to occur during labor and delivery. As you complete your plan, be prepared to tweak some of your preferences, as they could conflict with hospital policies. Together with your doula, your provider will help you reframe your expressed needs, wants, and desires by keeping them realistically flexible. Print several copies of your birth plan and present it with a basket of goodies to the health care team at the hospital (thanking them in advance for taking care of you and your newborn).

VAGINAL STEAMING

Vaginal steaming is the process of directing herb-infused steam into your vagina, usually by squatting over a container of hot liquid. It's known as the original women's health modality and can be ideal for labor preparation. Even though some women do this at home, it can be tricky to find the herbs that are right for you, not to mention the possibility of steam burns. Avoid any mishaps by going to a certified vaginal steam facilitator who will be able to prescribe the appropriate gentle blend and monitor the steam's intensity. Vaginal steaming is a safe, effective, noninvasive treatment that will let you move comfortably into labor feeling relaxed and uplifted. This treatment also helps prevent unnecessary medical interference, which will reduce the chances of birth trauma for mother and baby.

FREEZER MEALS

Late in the third trimester, pre-labor meal preparation can be stressful, so relax into the process. Make more food than you think you will need. Think "toddler food"—boneless and in chunks, so it's easy to eat one-handed—including about six weeks' worth of hearty snacks that you can eat with one hand and/or while standing. For comparison, that'd be the equivalent of making a quadruple batch of Oatmeal Lactation Cookies (page 152). Also, make it easier for friends and family to help you by freezing side dishes that will complement larger dishes. People looking to help tend to bring dinner meals, so stock your freezer with breakfast and lunchtime foods. However, you don't need to adhere to rules about *breakfast*, *lunch*, or *dinner* foods. Eat what you want. Do what you can and know that you cannot do it all.

FINANCIAL BUDGET

Like third-trimester meal prep, organizing a post-pregnancy budget can seem overwhelming. It takes some thought to figure out not only how to prepare but what to prepare *for*. Looking at the childrearing costs you may wonder if you can even afford the baby at all! Not to worry—with some maneuvering, a workable financial plan is totally doable.

Now is also a good time to draw up or update your will while you are clear-headed and have the time. Although creating a will won't be as much fun as putting together a baby registry, it is an essential part of becoming a parent and protecting your baby's future. If this is not the ideal time for you, give some thought to drafting a will as soon as possible so that you can ensure that your child is provided and cared for exactly how you desire. As baby takes center stage, you will need to make some upfront adjustments, temporarily putting some previous lifestyle habits aside. Breastfeeding eliminates the cost of bottles and formula while hand-me-downs keep your baby's clothing budget to a minimum. Let your friends and family know what you and your baby actually need. Otherwise, you will wind up with items in your nursery that you will never even use. Be practical.

FINISH THE NURSERY

One of the most satisfying moments of a pregnancy is putting the finishing touches on the nursery. Completing this task *before* week 33 lets you participate while you still have some mobility. Even though this is an intimate and personal project, let friends and family help you, especially with heavy lifting, assembling furniture, or painting. In part 1, we created a list of nursery items that commonly contain VOCs (see page 3). Take another look at this list when making decisions about the items you are using to decorate the nursery.

Hospital "Go-Bag" Checklists

Every expectant mom needs a packed bag ready to go for the hospital. Remember, there will be aspects of your delivery and birth plan that you can't control, but being as prepared as you can will go a long way toward peace of mind and a smooth delivery. Here are some essential items for your hospital go bag.

FOR LABOR AND DELIVERY

- CELL PHONE, the all-important item, serves as entertainment, a watch, camera, and video camera. Don't forget the charger!

- ENTERTAINMENT AND HOBBIES, including your laptop, tablet, playing cards, Sudoku or crossword puzzles, and knitting yarn will help you pass time and redirect your focus.

ESSENTIAL OILS (unscented or with your preferred scents) will be useful for lower back, foot, and/or hand massages, as well as on acupressure points.

EXTRA CLOTHES for your partner might be necessary, depending on the time and stage of labor you are in when you get to the hospital.

HAIR SUPPLIES, from combs and brushes to headbands and headscarves will definitely be needed. You may also want to have certain products available for maintenance.

JOURNAL AND PEN for note-taking regarding labor, delivery, and postpartum. You will also want to write down the staff's names, questions, and specific instructions.

MASSAGE BALL OR OTHER MASSAGE TOOL to adjust pressure will be useful for your doula or partner when hand massages are no longer effective.

PILLOWS with your own scent and tailored to your personal preferences (size, shape, color, and texture) will help you remain comfortable during labor and postpartum.

READING MATERIALS keep your mind actively engaged, although they might not get much use based on your labor stage when you arrive at the hospital.

SEVERAL COPIES OF YOUR BIRTH PLAN accompanied by a thoughtful gift for the health care team who will be taking care of you and your newborn. A little kindness goes a long way.

SLIPPERS that are comfortable, fit properly, and have nonskid grips on the soles are especially useful and specifically designed for your safety during the extended hallway walks during labor.

SNACKS, SANDWICHES, AND OTHER NONPERISHABLE LIGHT FARE for your partner (your doula will pack her own means of sustenance) will help them avoid missing important moments.

SOCKS that are soft, heavy, yet comfortable are another necessity, as hospital rooms are notoriously inadequately climate-controlled and usually on the colder side.

☐ SUGARLESS CANDY OR GUM will keep you from becoming parched and your mouth from drying out. Continue drinking small amounts of clear liquids during labor.

☐ TABLET OR SMARTPHONE so you can play soothing and relaxing music along with the extra special playlist you created especially for your baby's arrival.

☐ TIMER for monitoring contractions, like a stopwatch. Your partner and doula should also begin practicing timing your contractions during the last weeks of the third trimester.

☐ TOOTHBRUSH, TOOTHPASTE, AND MOUTHWASH are also necessities. You'll want to refresh your mouth and your breath after spending uninterrupted time confined in a hospital room.

FOR POSTPARTUM

☐ CONTACT INFORMATION for your closest friends and family is already in your phone but you should write down any numbers that aren't. Again, remember your phone charger!

☐ FEMININE HYGIENE PRODUCTS—sanitary napkins or period panties *not* menstrual cups or tampons—will be nice to have, even though the hospital provides pads for postpartum bleeding.

☐ GOING-HOME OUTFIT that fits as if you were about five to six months pregnant. Even though you are no longer pregnant, you're not quite ready for pre-pregnancy clothes.

☐ INFANT CAR SEAT that is properly installed *before* delivery. Without one, you may not legally be able to take your child home.

☐ PAJAMAS that are clean, well worn, and front opening are more comfortable than what the hospital offers. They'll make breastfeeding and skin-to-skin contact easily accessible, but bring an older pair since they'll probably get stained.

- SNACKS specific to your blood type, including trail mix and lactation cookies, will help keep you satisfied if hospital meals are unappealing.

- TOILETRIES, including a washcloth, soap, shampoo, conditioner, body wash, loofah, body towel, face cleanser, moisturizer, hand towel, body oil/lotion/creams, deodorant, makeup, and any other essentials, are all items you'll want after several hours (or a couple of days) in the hospital.

- UNDERGARMENTS (multiple changes of postpartum compression panties and a properly fitting nursing bra) don't need to be fancy but should be high waisted, comfortable, and supportive. A nice robe can help you feel more like yourself than what the hospital provides and will look better in all those pictures you'll be taking.

Braxton-Hicks Contractions

As your due date draws closer, you may begin to feel very mild contractions. These can be hardly perceptible or actually painful. You may also feel a slight tightness that begins at the top of your uterus and spreads downward, lasting from 15 seconds to 2 minutes. You may also feel discomfort in the groin, lower abdomen, or back. All these are versions of nonproductive contractions (false labor). Your body is getting ready—priming, practicing, and preparing for the productive contractions of labor that will thin and dilate (open) your cervix. Braxton-Hicks contractions are irregular in their timing and do not become more frequent or severe. If and when these contractions become uncomfortable, walk around or change position. Lie down if you have been standing, for example, or walk if you have been sitting.

Preparatory contractions are more regular and feel more like active labor contractions. They often occur in the afternoon or evening, after physical activity or sexual intercourse. They're also more likely to occur when you are tired and even mildly dehydrated, so be sure that you keep drinking water. Imagine these contractions are like a rehearsal for actual labor. Practice your breathing exercises and the other childbirth techniques you learned so that you can more effectively manage labor contractions. Begin timing and keeping a record of your contractions and how they feel. When the contractions do not subside with a change in activity and become progressively stronger

WHAT IS CORD BLOOD BANKING?

Cord blood is the blood left in the umbilical cord and placenta after your baby is born. It has been successfully used to treat childhood leukemia, some immune diseases, and some blood diseases.

Cord blood contains invaluable stem cells that are found in the bone marrow. These cells provide the foundation for the blood and immune systems. As these specialized cells are underdeveloped in the cord blood, they do not need to be matched (blood type and Rh factor) as closely for a transplant as bone marrow does. This feature is especially important for members of ethnic minority groups and people with rare blood types who have more difficulty finding acceptable donor matches.

Before your delivery, you may request that your baby's cord blood be collected and banked (frozen cryogenically and stored) for future use, either privately, for the use of your family only, or publicly, listed in a registry for patients all over the world. Public cord blood banking saves lives, is completely free, and includes collecting, testing, processing, and storage. The cost of private cord blood banking ranges between $1,400 and $2,300 for collection, testing, and registration, plus an additional yearly fee ranging between $95 and $125 for storage. Cord blood harvesting, a painless procedure that takes less than five minutes, is done after the umbilical cord has been clamped and cut. The procedure is safe for the mother and newborn as long as the cord is not prematurely clamped and cut.

and more regular, you may be in labor. Contact your provider if you have more than four nonproductive contractions (false labor contractions that do not progressively advance labor) in an hour.

Recipes for the Third Trimester

BREAKFAST

ITALIAN SAUSAGE, SWEET POTATO, AND CAULIFLOWER HASH

PROTEIN POWER, **VEGGIE LOADED**

SERVES 4 / PREP TIME: 10 MINUTES / COOK TIME: 30 MINUTES

Many women struggle with constipation during their third trimester. It is important to get in enough fiber from whole food sources to help prevent this. This recipe is a great breakfast option to start your day with a good amount of fiber, a little bit of protein, and a lot of flavor!

3 tablespoons extra-virgin olive oil, divided

1 medium sweet potato, shredded

½ head cauliflower, shredded

1 teaspoon dried rosemary

1 teaspoon dried thyme

½ teaspoon garlic powder

½ teaspoon sea salt

½ teaspoon black pepper

1 pound ground Italian sausage

1. Heat 2 tablespoons of olive oil in a sauté pan over medium-high heat. Add the sweet potato, cauliflower, rosemary, thyme, garlic powder, salt, and pepper.

2. Cook the vegetables until softened, about 10 minutes. Stir often to prevent any burning.

3. Heat the remaining 1 tablespoon of olive oil in a separate sauté pan on medium-high heat until hot, about 3 minutes.

4. Add the sausage and cook until no longer pink and heated through, about 10 minutes.

5. Divide the sweet potato–cauliflower hash among four plates and top each with 3 to 4 ounces of the sausage to serve.

PER SERVING: Calories: 524; Total fat: 41g; Saturated fat: 12g; Cholesterol: 81mg; Sodium: 1,508mg; Carbohydrates: 17g; Fiber: 3g; Protein: 24g

PREP TIP: If you want to add even more vegetables and protein, serve this dish along with a cooked egg and sautéed kale.

GOAT CHEESE CRANBERRY-WALNUT SALAD

QUICK AND EASY

SERVES 2 / PREP TIME: 10 MINUTES

Arugula is an amazing and tasty leafy green vegetable and forms the base of this salad. It pairs nicely with the walnuts, goat cheese, and cranberries. This is a simple salad with great flavor that will provide you and your developing baby with protein, good fats, and fiber to support your digestive system.

FOR THE DRESSING

3 tablespoons extra-virgin olive oil

1 tablespoon balsamic vinegar

¼ teaspoon sea salt

¼ teaspoon black pepper

1 teaspoon honey

FOR THE SALAD

4 cups arugula

2 ounces goat cheese

½ cup chopped walnuts

½ cup dried cranberries

TO MAKE THE DRESSING

1. In a small bowl, combine the olive oil, vinegar, salt, pepper, and honey, and mix well.

TO MAKE THE SALAD

2. Put the arugula in a large bowl and top with the goat cheese, walnuts, and cranberries.

3. Pour the dressing on top and toss gently to combine.

4. Serve the salad in two separate bowls.

PER SERVING: Calories: 623; Total fat: 48g; Saturated fat: 11g; Cholesterol: 15mg; Sodium: 430mg; Carbohydrates: 44g; Fiber: 5g; Protein: 12g

SUBSTITUTION TIP: Don't care for walnuts and/or cranberries? Swap the walnuts for sliced almonds or chopped pecans. Try raisins, apples, or dates instead of cranberries.

ASPARAGUS SHRIMP ONE-PAN MEAL

PROTEIN POWER

SERVES 4 / PREP TIME: 15 MINUTES / COOK TIME: 30 MINUTES

This meal brings perfect balance to your third-trimester needs with a green vegetable, healthy protein, and a starchy vegetable. One-pan meals are great for their simplicity and minimal clean-up. Shrimp is an excellent protein source that is lower in mercury content.

4 medium red potatoes, sliced

3 tablespoons extra-virgin olive oil, divided

1½ teaspoons sea salt, divided

½ teaspoon garlic powder

1 pound asparagus, woody ends removed

1 teaspoon black pepper, divided

1 pound large raw shrimp

½ teaspoon red pepper flakes

½ cup chopped fresh parsley

1. Preheat the oven to 375°F.
2. Toss the potato slices in a large bowl with 1 tablespoon of olive oil, ½ teaspoon of salt, and garlic powder.
3. Spread the potatoes out on a baking sheet. Bake for 10 minutes.
4. While the potatoes are cooking, put the asparagus in a large bowl and toss with 1 tablespoon of olive oil, ½ teaspoon of salt, and ½ teaspoon of pepper.
5. Toss the shrimp in a separate bowl with the remaining 1 tablespoon of olive oil, remaining ½ teaspoon of salt, remaining ½ teaspoon of pepper, and the red pepper flakes.
6. Pull the baking sheet out of the oven, flip the potatoes, then add the asparagus. Bake for 13 minutes.
7. Pull the baking sheet out, add the shrimp, and bake for 6 to 7 minutes until cooked through.
8. Top with fresh parsley and serve.

PER SERVING: Calories: 346; Total fat: 11g; Saturated fat: 2g; Cholesterol: 180mg; Sodium: 1,562mg; Carbohydrates: 40g; Fiber: 6g; Protein: 24g

SUBSTITUTION TIP: If you do not prefer your foods even a little spicy, you can omit the red pepper flakes. You can swap the red potatoes for sweet potatoes, too.

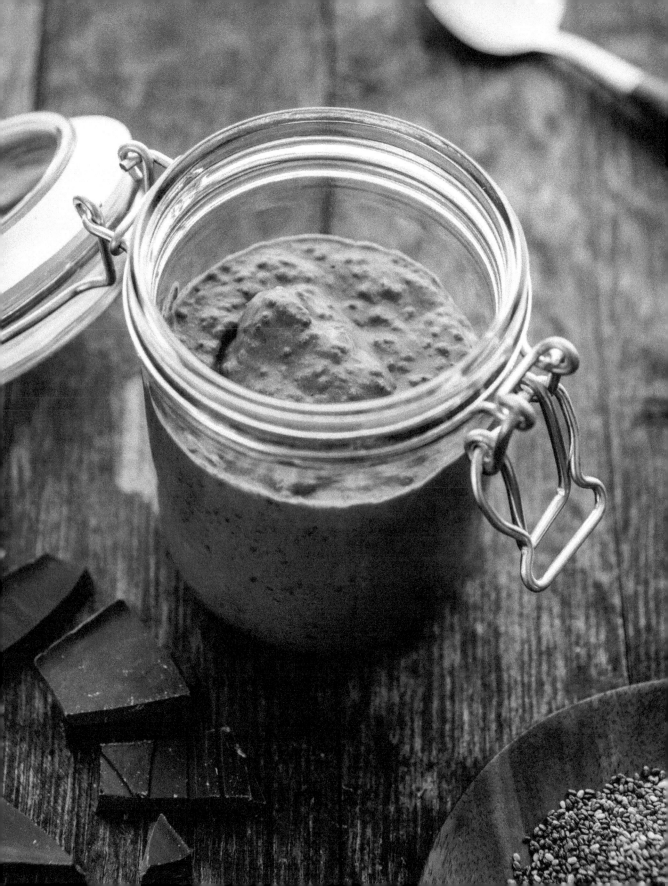

CHOCOLATE CHIA-SEED PUDDING

LABOR SUPPORTIVE, QUICK AND EASY

SERVES 6 / PREP TIME: 5 MINUTES, PLUS AT LEAST 3 HOURS TO CHILL

This sweet treat is perfect for the third trimester of pregnancy. It is packed with fiber to help prevent constipation and includes dates, which are said to help support an easier labor. It's a perfect, guilt-free dessert made from quality ingredients to help nourish your body.

1½ cups canned coconut milk

1 tablespoon cocoa powder

¼ teaspoon sea salt

6 dates

1 teaspoon vanilla extract

3 tablespoons chia seeds

1. Put the coconut milk, cocoa powder, salt, dates, vanilla extract, and chia seeds in a blender. Blend well.

2. Pour into a storage container. Let chill for at least 3 hours or overnight before serving.

PER SERVING: Calories: 156; Total fat: 12g; Saturated fat: 9g; Cholesterol: 0mg; Sodium: 104mg; Carbohydrates: 11g; Fiber: 4g; Protein: 2g

SUBSTITUTION TIP: Try swapping the vanilla extract for peppermint extract to make this into a chocolate-mint pudding. Reduce the amount of dates if you want it less sweet.

RASPBERRY-LEAF THIRD-TRIMESTER SUPPORT SMOOTHIE

LABOR SUPPORTIVE, LIGHT BITE, QUICK AND EASY
SERVES 1 / PREP TIME: 5 MINUTES

This smoothie is delicious and simple. It includes dates and red raspberry leaf tea, which are said to be beneficial during your third trimester to help prepare and support the body during labor. The dates also provide fiber and give a perfect, natural sweetness to this beverage. The celery and berries add more nutrition and fiber.

1 cup raspberry leaf tea

1 cup frozen mixed berries

1 medium celery stalk

3 dates

1. Brew raspberry leaf tea (either loose leaf or tea bag) according to package instructions. Let it cool to room temperature or refrigerate.
2. Put the tea, berries, celery, and dates into a blender. Blend well and serve immediately.

PER SERVING: Calories: 136; Total fat: <1g; Saturated fat: 0g; Cholesterol: 0mg; Sodium: 47mg; Carbohydrates: 34g; Fiber: 5g; Protein: 2g

PREP TIP: You can modify the number of dates based on how sweet you would like this smoothie. Try substituting cucumber for the celery to get in a different vegetable.

Essential Oil Blends for the Third Trimester

This section contains essential oil blends designed to alleviate some common ailments you may encounter during the third trimester.

DRY SKIN

Dry skin still an issue in the third trimester? Try Chamomile essential oil to soothe the skin while reducing the itchiness associated with dryness. Combine 5 to 10 drops of Chamomile oil to almond carrier oil and apply it directly to your body right after showering but before you dry off. You can also use Evening Primrose essential oil, which contains essential fatty acids needed to keep your skin tissue healthy. Lavender essential oil is also an excellent choice for dry skin moisturizing. Rose Geranium essential oil can also help dry skin, especially when combined with other essential oils, such as the Lavender and/or Chamomile.

HEMORRHOIDS

If hemorrhoids are still flaring up, try this combination to ease hemorrhoidal pain and inflammation. Combine six drops of Cypress, three drops of Myrtle, and three drops of German Chamomile essential oils with one ounce of St. John's Wort carrier oil, and apply externally. For more healing and protection, heat the carrier oil and add ½ teaspoon of shaved beeswax *before* adding the essential oils. You can also add two drops of Frankincense essential oil to constrict distended veins. If you have broken skin, apply a compress of Carrot Seed essential oil, made by soaking a cloth in water and adding three drops of the oil.

REFLUX/INDIGESTION

We've already talked about reflux caused by indigestion and your ever-expanding uterus. In addition to those factors, poor digestion can also result from the improper breakdown of proteins. To counteract this, gently massage your abdomen with a combination of five drops of Chamomile essential oil, three drops of Dill essential oil, two drops of Ginger essential oil, two drops of Peppermint essential oil, and one ounce of your preferred carrier oil to soothe your stomach. Due to the size of your uterus, your stomach may not be at your navel, so apply accordingly. You can also add Juniper Berry and Black Pepper essential oils to the essential oil blend.

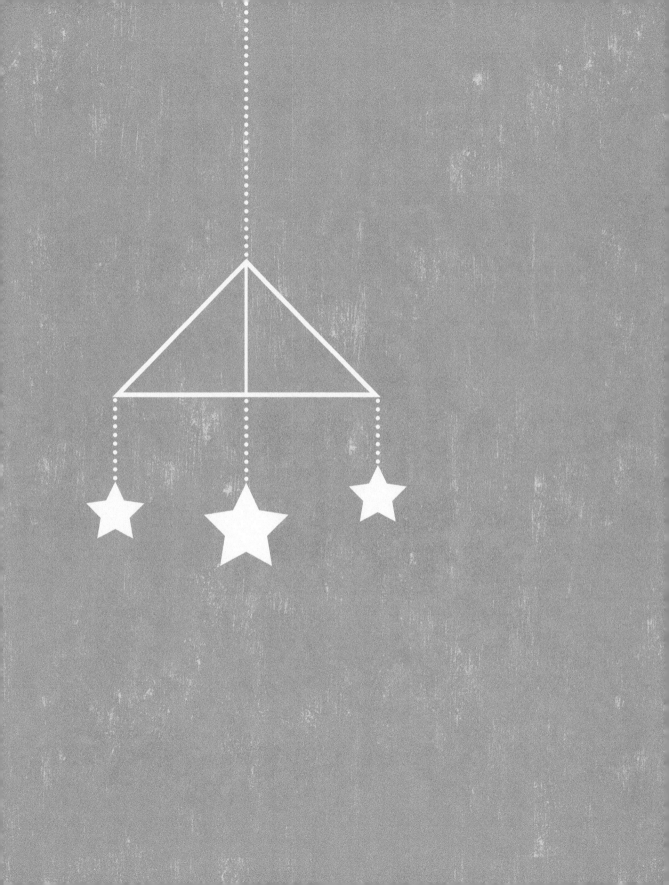

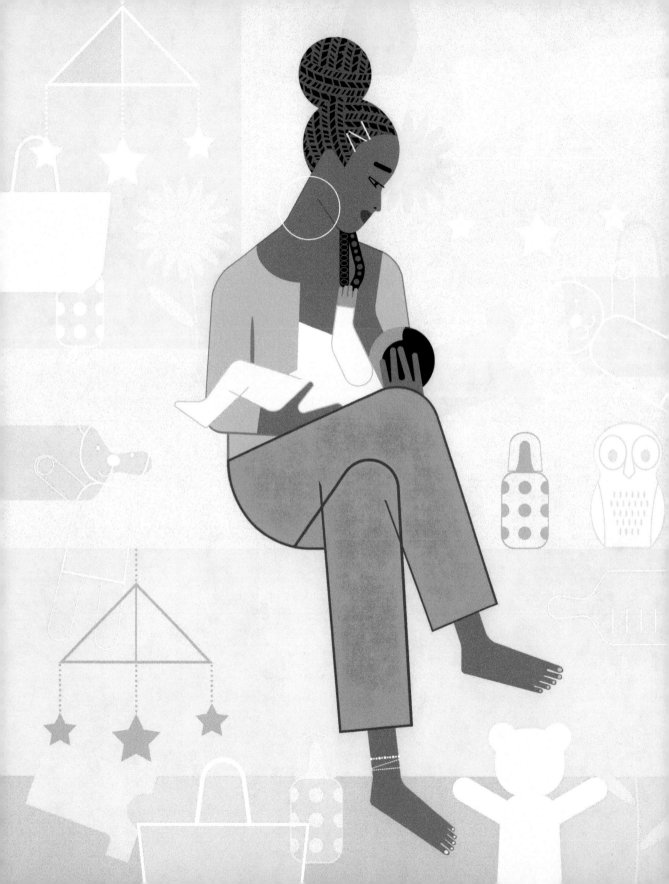

Part Three

BIRTH AND BEYOND

Opting to have a traditional hospital birth (or being advised to do so) may require some flexibility; however, it doesn't have to completely derail your delivery plans. Committing to a nonmedicated, chemical-free postpartum period is worth the effort, as it helps both your newborn and your emotional recovery. Consider your newborn as a fetus growing *outside* the womb during this time. The "fourth trimester," the first three months of a newborn's life, will be filled with your baby's fussiness and crying coupled with your exhaustion, stress, and frustration. Many mothers underestimate the wide-ranging physical and emotional demands of the postpartum period. For this reason, coming up with a strategy for your evolving provider team, which by now can include a physician or midwife, an acupuncturist, a postpartum doula, a pelvic floor physical therapist, and a lactation support consultant, is one of the best practical decisions you can make. You'll also learn through trial and error which calming techniques soothe your baby. It's demanding, which is why all that preparation (did you make your frozen snacks?) was so important.

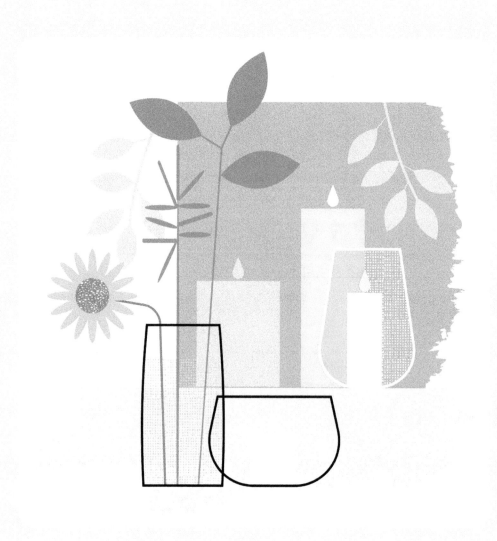

CHAPTER SEVEN

An Unmedicated Birth

Choosing to have an unmedicated birth experience seems like an obvious decision; however, it can be quite challenging. It requires an ongoing commitment (barring unforeseen circumstances). If you can, take a class to learn more about unmedicated birth. Get your intentions on the record by telling your health care provider, nurse, partner, and family about the details. Mothers-to-be with this level of active, built-in support during delivery are one step closer to ensuring their birth goes according to their preferences.

Unmedicated childbirth not only feels different for the mother, but it also *looks* different from the provider's perspective. Providers who advocate for unmedicated births work well with midwives and doulas, use minimal interventions, and have lower cesarean birth rates. As you learn what to expect, and as labor progresses, explore the ways that you experience comfort (through meditation, music, prayer, etc.) within yourself. Ask specific questions about the pain so that you will be prepared for it. Whether you have a midwife, doula, or a supportive partner, the most important factor is trust. With slower, more manageable contractions, relaxing will help your body do its job more effectively and efficiently. If you get overwhelmed or emotional, your labor support personnel will help you remain calm, relaxed, and engaged in the process. You being engaged and really feeling the contractions will yield unparalleled oxytocin and adrenaline-sponsored relief when your baby emerges from your body. Have faith in yourself and believe you can do this. You can.

Birth Centers vs. Hospitals vs. Home Births

Think of birthing centers as a hybrid option for low-risk pregnancies. They're kind of a middle ground between hospitals and home births. They are usually standalone facilities that let you have your prenatal appointments, childbirth and breastfeeding classes, and unmedicated birth all under one roof. They are popular but scarce, so finding one may be difficult. Many insurance plans don't cover birthing centers, so check your policy before making commitments. Out-of-pocket costs for birthing centers can be $10,000 or more.

However, unlike most hospitals, birthing centers offer a personalized touch. They have private rooms, soft lighting, showers, jacuzzi tubs, and a kitchen available for family. Located minutes from hospitals (in case of emergency or a needed epidural), birthing centers are staffed by midwives and on-call obstetricians. Generally, birthing centers use only low-level interventions, such as intravenous therapy, oxygen therapy, and infant resuscitation, and no fetal monitoring. Birthing centers carry less risk than home births, which are only available for low-risk births. Home births require you to get a physician or certified nurse midwife, have available transportation, and live within 10 to 15 miles of the nearest hospital.

QUESTIONS TO ASK WHEN TOURING A BIRTHING CENTER

Is it licensed by the state where you plan to deliver and accredited by the Commission for the Accreditation of Birth Centers?

Are the majority of the midwives who practice there credentialed as certified nurse-midwives, certified midwives, or certified professional midwives?

How many years of total birth center experience does this location have, and which doctor(s) provide backup in case of emergency situations beyond your scope of practice?

Do they offer classes such as childbirth education, newborn care, breastfeeding, and postpartum adjustment? What community referrals and resources are available?

How are "high-risk" pregnancies managed, and in which circumstances does a physician become the provider during pregnancy and labor/delivery?

Do the midwives provide continuous support during labor, and if not, does it have experience with doulas during labor and delivery?

What are your policies and practices about intravenous therapy during labor, activity and movement, eating and drinking during labor, and traditional positioning during delivery?

What is the standard approach if labor is progressing slowly? How will you monitor the well-being of my baby during labor without fetal monitoring?

How should I prepare for managing pain during labor and delivery? Besides nitrous oxide, what unmedicated measures and techniques for pain relief are available?

What complications in delivery or postpartum will require me to transfer to a hospital? Which hospital would I use if a transfer becomes necessary?

Are providers certified in neonatal resuscitation? What kind of resuscitation equipment is available? Under what circumstances would my baby be transferred to a hospital?

What percentage of births involve an emergency transfer during labor? After labor? What percentage end in a cesarean delivery? What percentage of newborns are subsequently hospitalized?

If my baby is healthy, will providers facilitate skin-to-skin contact immediately after delivery? Are there instances that require our immediate separation after delivery?

How long is the postpartum stay and what type of instruction will I receive with breastfeeding? Will this assistance continue after my discharge?

What services are included in the fees and associated costs for maternal care? Do you accept insurance and what other payment arrangements are available?

QUESTIONS TO ASK WHEN TOURING A HOSPITAL

When should I come to the hospital? Where do I first go when I am in labor? Is there a specific maternity care entrance?

Will students or residents participate (peripherally or directly) in the delivery? How do I communicate my wishes if I am uncomfortable with this arrangement?

Describe the labor and delivery rooms. Are they all the same? How do they differ? Are labor and delivery rooms private or shared?

What amenities are included in each room? Does each room have a refrigerator? A birthing tub? Will staff allow delivery in a water-filled tub?

How many pillows are there in each room? How many am I allowed to have? May I request more or should I bring my own?

How often do doulas attend births at this hospital? Is there a bed, cot, or specified sleeping area for my doula and my partner?

My desire is for an unmedicated, intervention-free labor and delivery. How will the hospital care team facilitate my desires to execute my birth plans?

What are the policies regarding eating and drinking during labor? What food options will be available and what will I be able to eat?

Are there different food options for my partner and doula? Is there a cafeteria? What time does the cafeteria close? Are there vending machines?

What is the visitor policy? How many visitors are allowed during labor, delivery, and postpartum? What are the visiting hours for these time periods?

Is my partner allowed in the operating room for a cesarean delivery? Will my doula be able to facilitate breastfeeding immediately after cesarean delivery?

Is there an international board-certified lactation consultant on staff? What are the hours? How do I access this person if I deliver during the weekend?

Is this hospital designated as "baby-friendly"? Are pacifiers given to babies? Will my baby "room-in" with me or will they stay in the nursery?

Do the newborn procedures include delayed cord clamping? How do I donate our cord blood? How is the first hour after birth typically managed?

What does the procedure involve for taking the placenta home with me? What documentation is needed and what materials do I need for transport?

WATER BIRTH

Water birth, delivering underwater to simulate the environment of the womb, is an uncommon practice in the contemporary medical community. Regardless, it is a gentle birth option. As a baby eases from the warm, liquid environment of the womb into another warm, liquid environment it feels a familiar comfort after the stress of passing through the birth canal. After delivery, the provider pulls the newborn from the water and immediately places her skin-to-skin on the mother's chest. Partners can join the mother in the tub or portable birthing pool by actively supporting her from behind.

Most women with low-risk pregnancies can opt for a water birth if they can get a willing and licensed practitioner and adequate facilities to host the delivery. Birthing centers are more equipped to offer this option. Water births are usually performed at home and in birthing centers, rarely in hospitals. Unfortunately, if your pregnancy is high risk, you may not be eligible for water delivery. You may also have challenges locating a midwife willing to attend a delivery that is already perceived as higher risk due to lack of research. If you are unable to proceed with a water birth, try to labor in a whirlpool tub or warm-water bathtub as long as possible so you can enjoy the relaxation, pain relief, and gravity-free environment that moves labor along.

Your Birth Team

Building your birth team will be one of the most important steps you take as you prepare for labor and delivery. Assembling a team of practitioners to assist in your plan for an unmedicated, intervention-less labor and delivery should begin immediately. It may be challenging to make substantial changes in the second or third trimester, so start as early as possible. This is a personal process for you and your family. Finances, as always, will be a factor. Begin by choosing a provider that aligns with your personal birth philosophy, your goals, and your desires. A birth doula who provides labor support will be an excellent addition to your team; however, a supportive person (preferably not your partner) who is knowledgeable of your preferences can be helpful as well. Your team does not have to be large in number. It just needs to be large in constructive support as the team members embrace you physically and emotionally.

First, consider the environment where you'll feel the most comfortable delivering, whether it's at home, in a birth center, or in a hospital. During this time, you will want to ask *all* your questions, interview multiple practitioners and professionals, and connect with potential members of your ideal birth team. When deciding who to have on your team, consider the people with whom you feel most comfortable and the people who share your birthing philosophies. Ensuring that you have a team to support you (literally and figuratively) through the process of labor and delivery is important to having a positive birth experience.

Your support team may consist of a primary support layperson (spouse/ partner, close family member, or friend) in addition to practitioners (doula, massage therapist, vaginal steam facilitator, pelvic floor physical therapist, acupuncturist, yoga instructor, nutritionist, health coach, and/or clinical herbalist), and professionals (midwife, obstetrician, or family physician who will support your birth plan preferences). This section will highlight the differences between doulas and midwives while providing a list of questions to ask when interviewing them.

DOULAS

An increasing number of mothers-to-be choose to hire a birth doula, a labor support companion who takes some of the pressure off their partner during long and/or intense labor. The services a doula provides depend on the type of doula you have selected, at what point in your pregnancy you hire your doula, and your overall preferences. Women supported by doulas are less likely to need cesarean sections, induction, and pain medication; they also tend to have shorter labor with fewer complications. Depending on your preferences, your doula can assist with the design of your birth plan, ease your pre-labor anxiety, and help you through early labor at home before going to the birthing facility.

The doula is there to be a constant source of comfort, encouragement, and emotional and physical support during labor. Your doula will be a calming voice of experience providing relaxation techniques, breathing exercises, and advice on labor positions. She will also be an advocate, translating medical terminology and explaining procedures as needed. Throughout labor and delivery, your doula will be the only person (besides your partner) who will be by your side from beginning to end. Postpartum doulas offer support after delivery ranging from breastfeeding to baby care and errands to light housework. Overall, the doula will be a cooperative member of your labor support team who is ready to offer support without being overbearing.

QUESTIONS WHEN INTERVIEWING A DOULA

Why did you originally decide to become a doula?

Tell me about your training and why you chose it.

Through what organization or entity are you certified?

How many births have you attended?

How would you describe your doula style?

What is your pricing structure and what does it include?

After the birth, do you meet with me to discuss labor, review delivery, and answer questions?

What happens if you are with another client when I go into labor? Who will support me?

Who is your backup doula and when can we meet?

How did you choose your backup doula?

When will you be on call for my delivery?

How will you support my partner/family member/birthing coach?

Will you supply me with references I can contact and/or reviews I can read?

Do you offer any additional services like hypnobirthing, placenta encapsulation, and/or birth photography?

How many other clients do you have around my due date?

Describe your relationship or previous interactions with my provider/hospital staff.

What happens if my birth goes differently than I anticipated? How do you help me adjust?

What do you carry in your doula bag?

QUESTIONS FOR YOU

Do you feel like your doula(s) listened to you? Did they ask you any questions? Were they interested in you and what you desire from your birth experience?

Do you feel like you clicked with them?

MIDWIVES

Certified nurse-midwives (CNMs) are medical professionals, registered nurses certified by the American College of Nurse-Midwives, who receive special graduate-school-level training in the field of midwifery. A CNM is trained to care for women with low-risk pregnancies throughout labor and uncomplicated deliveries. During the postpartum period, they often provide routine gynecological care and newborn care. Midwives emphasize whole-woman care by giving you time to discuss your emotional well-being alongside your physical recovery. With a midwife, you will receive nutritional advice, health coaching, and breastfeeding support. Most important, midwives are more experienced, and more inclined and better oriented toward an unmedicated, intervention-less labor and delivery.

Most CNMs work in hospital settings or deliver at birthing centers; however, direct-entry midwives are more likely to attend home births. Direct-entry midwives are midwives who are trained without becoming nurses, though they may hold degrees in other areas of health care. Direct-entry midwives who receive their certification through the North American Registry of Midwives are certified professional midwives (CPMs). In most states, midwives are authorized to offer epidurals and other forms of pain relief, and prescribe labor-inducing medications; however, deliveries attended by midwives are much less likely to include these types of interventions. Because they only care for women with low-risk pregnancies, midwives have much lower cesarean delivery rates than physicians. Prenatal care costs associated with a CNM are less than those of physicians, though many CNMs work with qualified physicians for backup support in complicated cases and special-care referrals.

QUESTIONS WHEN INTERVIEWING A MIDWIFE

What inspired you to become a midwife?

How does your practice operate?

Describe how prenatal care with a midwife looks and feels different than with a physician.

Will a student midwife be involved in my care?

How do you support women with varied cultural beliefs and religious traditions surrounding birth?

What happens if there's a complication in my pregnancy?

When am I considered overdue and what happens then?

Who will be allowed to support me during labor and delivery?

What kind of mobility is allowed?

Can you describe what happens during labor and birth?

Am I eligible for a home delivery or delivery at a birthing center?

What partnerships do you have with physicians, institutions where I might be transferred, and other organizations with which I (or my baby) may need assistance?

What will our interactions look like when early labor begins?

How are my baby and I cared for postpartum?

Do you support an undisturbed delivery philosophy?

Are there interventions that are a part of your standard protocol?

In what instances are interventions absolutely necessary?

What coping mechanisms will you offer to help me avoid unnecessary interventions?

Will you be able to assist me with breastfeeding?

Based on where you attend births, what restrictions might be placed on me because of protocol?

Your Birth Plan Checklist

Think about it: what do you want your birth experience to look like? Following a birth plan for an unmedicated, intervention-free labor and delivery requires time and intentional preparation on your behalf. Thinking about your preferences and weighing your options early in your pregnancy while adjusting *throughout* your pregnancy is a key step, not only in making a plan but in carrying it out. Hiring a doula and taking at least one childbirth class will ensure that you are prepared and that, regardless of your preferences, you'll be able to adjust. Familiarizing yourself with nonmedicated pain management techniques and interventions will also be beneficial.

Here are some items you'll want to consider when making your birth plan:

ATMOSPHERE. What will help you feel most comfortable. Dimmed lights? Soft, classical music in the background? A quiet room? A closed door? A limited number of guests? Candid photos being taken?

EPISIOTOMY. This intervention should not be taken lightly, as it affects your recovery. Include in your birth plan how you intend to prevent tearing (extra-virgin olive oil, coached or instinctive pushing, specific pushing positions, perineal support, and/or compresses). You might consider it, only if necessary, for the newborn's safety, allowing for natural tearing.

FOOD AND DRINK. Often this preference is only an option if your practitioner and/or birth location approves, but you may be able to drink or eat light foods during labor.

FORCEPS (OR VACUUM EXTRACTION). These instruments are designed to "guide" your newborn out of the birth canal during delivery. The use of forceps (and vacuum extraction) are risky for the mother and newborn and are rarely an absolute necessity.

FREE MOVEMENT. Is being able to walk around freely important to you? Do you want to be able to use a birthing ball? Would you like to be able to take a warm shower or bath? Have a clear understanding of what the birthing facility's capabilities are in terms of fetal monitoring (wireless monitoring and intermittent versus continuous), as this may affect your options.

GENTLE CESAREAN. If a C-section is absolutely necessary for your health and the health of your baby, you still have options. To initiate a family-centered cesarean delivery, walk yourself into the operating room, if possible, as this is an empowering act. Request that two support people accompany you in the operating room so that one person can welcome your baby while you still have support with you by your head. If you are waiting to discover the sex of your baby, you can still do that; the surgeons do not need to make this announcement. You can request a cord-clamping delay (even for a very short time) if your baby is stable. You can also ask that the drape be lowered at delivery so that you can see your baby.

Some hospitals that routinely practice gentle cesareans will bring your baby to your chest immediately after birth, allowing you and your baby to have immediate skin-to-skin contact. If this isn't possible, consider letting your partner (or designated person) have some skin-to-skin time with the baby right there in the OR. To prepare for a vaginal birth after cesarean (VBAC) attempt in a future pregnancy, ask for double-layer uterine suturing, as some physicians are more likely to consider a VBAC attempt if the uterus has been repaired in this way. When you get back to your room, start bonding with your baby and initiating breastfeeding with minimal distractions and visitors.

INDUCTION. This intervention moves labor along at a faster pace than occurs naturally, which may affect the recovery process. If induction is absolutely necessary, using a small uterine catheter called a Foley bulb is a medication-free option.

INTRAVENOUS FLUIDS. Specifically indicate in your birth plan if you want to accept routine IV fluids or an IV saline lock. Pre-labor hydration is important so be mindful of this throughout your pregnancy.

LABORING AT HOME AS LONG AS POSSIBLE. There will be pain and, in this scenario, arriving at the hospital later is better than arriving too early. You have prepared for this with birthing classes and your doula will guide you. Instead of an epidural or Pitocin, you will be going directly to the delivery room.

MEMBRANE SWEEPING. Recommended to promote spontaneous labor, to avoid prolonged pregnancy, and to reduce the need to be induced, membrane sweeping is often given without consent. To avoid this, be clear about your preferences, including nipple stimulation and/or movement.

NATURAL WATER RUPTURE. Specify that you would like to wait for this to happen on its own without instrumentation, if that's your preference.

☐ **A *PAID* DOULA OR LABOR SUPPORT PRACTITIONER.** Even though partners, parents, siblings, and friends are all great to have as a part of your support circle, they are not trained professionals. Having a trained professional with whom you feel comfortable giving you guidance specifically designed to enhance your birth experience is the way to go.

☐ **PAIN MANAGEMENT.** Do you want pain management to be available to you? Think about whether you want providers to *ask* you about employing pain control options, such as nitrous oxide (laughing gas), which is an analgesic, not anesthesia. As you design your birth plan, ask your provider (and your doula) about pain-relief options, as well as any questions you have about specific options like breathing, hypno-birthing, massage, heat therapy, and positioning.

☐ **A SUPPORTIVE PARTNER.** Even if you are a single mother-to-be, have a member of your support circle, someone who understands the specifics of your dream birth and can be with you for loving glances, moral support, and familiarity.

☐ **A SUPPORTIVE PRACTICE.** Whether you have a midwife or a physician, your provider needs to understand your vision of labor and delivery and be 100 percent on your team. Asking your provider specific questions regarding interventions, water-breaking time schedules, and due dates early on in your pregnancy will give you enough time to prepare, and to switch providers if necessary.

☐ **VAGINAL EXAMINATIONS.** Unnecessary vaginal examinations only increase your newborn's risk of infection. In addition, the disappointment can negatively work against your psyche if you are not progressing as quickly as you hoped. However, three well-spaced vaginal exams, performed by the same provider on arrival at the hospital and again a few hours later, are sufficient.

PITOCIN

Oxytocin is the natural hormone that triggers contractions and makes them stronger. Sold under the brand name Pitocin as a synthetic medication and labor stimulator, it is a common intervention used to induce contractions, speed up labor, and stop postpartum bleeding. During labor, your doctor may try administering prostaglandins (hormones that help ripen the cervix), stripping the membranes (sweeping the inside of your cervix), and/or artificially rupturing your membranes. If none of these things brings on regular contractions, your provider may give you Pitocin intravenously. While this is happening, your baby will be monitored to see how it responds to the contractions. If labor stalls, there *must* be an intervention of some kind in order to avoid sepsis or severe infection, otherwise the baby's life (and yours) could be in danger.

Pitocin has some risks. It can bring contractions too close together, not allowing enough time for the uterus to relax and recover, causing fetal distress. Women who are given Pitocin have an increased risk of having a baby with a lower Apgar score; their babies are also more likely to be admitted to the NICU. You also risk water intoxication (excessive water intake that pushes your electrolyte balance out of whack), pulmonary edema (excess fluid in the lungs), and abnormal sodium levels. Also, once your provider administers Pitocin you won't be able to eat or drink because of the increased risk of a cesarean delivery. If Pitocin is recommended, have your doula ask what the indications (valid reasons to use Pitocin) are and if there are any reasonable alternatives.

Natural Pain Relief

Knowing how to manage unmedicated labor is the most visceral challenge you'll encounter. Saying you do not want an epidural is easy; staying committed to that decision while dealing with back and abdominal pain is difficult. Having a clearly written birth plan in place along with a strong and supportive birth team will help you as you navigate the mental and physical effort that labor brings. If you are open to using medical pain relief, be sure to tell your doula and midwife that you would like to know when you get to the stage at which medical intervention is no longer an option. Then, at that point, you can ask what the indications are and decide on natural or medical pain relief.

If you are staying the course with an unmedicated, intervention-free labor, there are several options that can help ease the perception of pain during the labor and delivery process. If you ultimately decide to have medical intervention as labor progresses, nonmedication pain relief techniques can help you stay comfortable.

Pain relief during labor is approached in many ways. Decide before you go into labor which method will be the best for you. Also know your available options and which of those you would like to explore during labor and delivery. A clear pain management strategy will include a combination of methods.

BREATHING

For women experiencing contractions and hoping to avoid medication, breathing is a beneficial way to relieve tension without stalling labor. Lamaze, the oldest technique of childbirth preparation, emphasizes relaxation and breathing during labor and delivery. It teaches mothers to make their efforts fruitful during labor, rather than unproductive. Many midwives also suggest rhythmic breathing to encourage relaxation. Taking long, deep, slow, and steady breaths will ease labor pain. Do not be afraid to make moaning noises! Take deep breaths and let it all out through your mouth. Feel free to be as loud as you like. Breathing is fundamental.

ACUPUNCTURE AND ACUPRESSURE

Acupuncture can stimulate labor progress and can be an effective pain-relieving technique during active labor. In the weeks leading up to labor, you can safely receive acupuncture from a licensed acupuncturist experienced in treating pregnant women. Acupressure uses the same principles as acupuncture except, instead of using needles, the practitioner uses pressure applied with her fingers to stimulate the same points. Targeting strategic points throughout the body can help ease the discomfort and pain associated with labor. Before you try either one, talk to your provider and your doula.

REFLEXOLOGY

Like acupuncture and acupressure, reflexology accesses internal organs through specific points on your feet. Massaging specific pressure points in your feet throughout labor and delivery relaxes the uterus and stimulates the pituitary gland, which reduces pain and shortens labor. Although reflexology is not designed to induce labor, applying pressure to certain points on the feet can stimulate contractions, so reflexology can be a good alternative to medical induction. Before using reflexology for labor induction, make sure that the reflexologist is specifically trained to use it for this purpose.

HYPNOBIRTHING

Hypnosis enables you to achieve a state of concentration, deep relaxation, and focus, which can help relieve labor pain. Many women seek out clinically certified hypnotherapists to train them to self-hypnotize through labor and delivery. Some doulas also offer this as a part of their services, but it really requires consistent practice *during* pregnancy to get to the level of relaxation that enables you to be unaware of labor pain. During hypnobirthing, you are completely awake and aware of baby's arrival without any negative side effects for you or your newborn.

ACTIVITY

Contrary to conventional hospital practices, reclining on your back is the absolute worst position for pain management; it actually stalls labor progress. Changing positions as necessary lets you use your own body to adjust to your baby's movement through the birth canal. Walking and standing up also allows gravity to do its thing and aid in your baby's descent. Stand up, lean on the back of a chair, or slow dance with your partner for additional support. Positions like sitting on a birthing ball, straddling a chair, and resting on all fours rocking back and forth with your legs spread apart also open up your pelvis to help bring your newborn into the world.

MASSAGE

Massage can be a great way to ease labor pain. Try applying intense counter-pressure on your sore areas with knuckles, the heel of the hand, or a tennis ball coupled with hot compresses. Now is the time for your partner (or doula) to step up with some tension-relieving, muscle-relaxing head, back, and foot massages. Let your massage therapist manipulate your muscles and apply pressure in ways that help you relax while promoting oxygen flow. The scent of a preferred essential oil may be beneficial during a massage. If possible, lie on your left side during your massage to keep adequate blood flow to the placenta and to your baby.

HYDROTHERAPY

Even if you are unable to have a water birth, a warm bath in a whirlpool or hydrotherapy tub can help reduce pain as the jets knead your lower back. If your room has a shower, take advantage of the removable shower head's warm pulsations. Immersion hydrotherapy works beautifully once labor is well-established (four to five centimeters dilated with regular contractions), as it enables buoyant movement and relaxation during (and between) contractions. It helps cervical dilation and lowers blood pressure and, perhaps just as important, it gives you a sense of control and security.

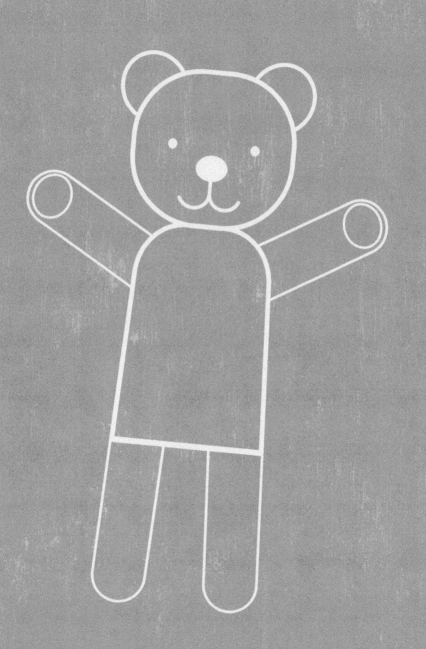

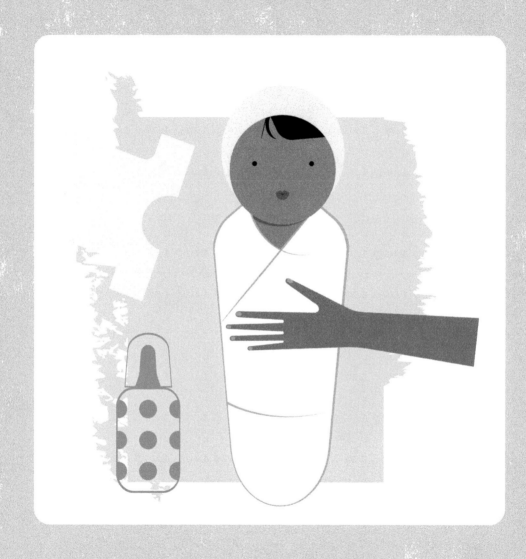

CHAPTER EIGHT

A Healthy, Wholesome Newborn

Welcoming your newborn into your life is a magical event, accompanied by a daunting number of things to remember to do. As soon as possible after birth, have skin-to-skin contact with your newborn. If you delivered in a hospital, ask that all newborn procedures be delayed until after your baby has nursed for the first time. Include it in your birth plan if necessary.

Your pregnancy does not end with the birth. There are a host of postpartum decisions to make to avoid unnecessary medical interventions being thrust upon your baby. This added stress can be overwhelming. Fear of the unknown is common and quite understandable, especially when coupled with exhaustion. You're going to be bombarded with information from the Internet, neighbors, family, and everyone else you meet. Don't take everything to heart. Avoiding information overload will help reduce your confusion, anxiety, and uncertainty.

There are a myriad of treatments that can occur immediately after delivery, such as umbilical cord management, circumcision, and vaccination. In addition, newborn and infant care at home will be much different than it was during your hospital stay. This chapter is designed to help you make decisions about the healthiest ways to feed, bathe, and bond with your baby as you ease into the first few weeks of life with your infant. Have confidence in yourself as a new parent. You've got this!

The After-Delivery Checklist

After delivery, your birth plan (free of medication and interventions) requires preparation, awareness, focus, and continuous communication with your health care team. While there are several options in the following list, be thoughtful and consider them carefully. The knowledge will empower you, especially in the moment, and help reduce your anxiety about what's best for you and your baby. Think about how you want the moments after your baby's arrival to unfold. What are your postpartum expectations? Be sure to have additional copies of the postpartum/after-delivery portion of your birth plan available for new shift members. Remember your ultimate goal—a healthy baby and a healthy YOU.

- BATHING. Newborns are born with vernix, a white coating with protective, temperature-regulating, and germ-fighting properties. Consider it an emollient that you can rub into their skin. You can delay your baby's first bath past the hospital stay until you are at home and feel ready. Ideally, bathing should be delayed until after 24 hours of birth. If this is not possible for cultural reasons, it should be delayed for at least eight hours in order to reduce the instability associated with cold stress.

- BREASTFEEDING. To breastfeed exclusively, include "no formula, sugar water, pacifiers, or bottles" in your postpartum plan. Facilities that are "baby friendly" are great about supporting this preference.

- CIRCUMCISION. Vitamin K is essential for blood clotting. If you opt for circumcision, waiting until your newborn's own vitamin K production begins (around the eighth day of life) is a wise choice.

CORD CUTTING. Do you want someone other than the health care team to cut the umbilical cord? Remember that delayed cord clamping will delay the ceremonial cord cutting.

DELAYED CORD CLAMPING. Before the umbilical cord stops pulsating and turns white, it delivers oxygen-rich blood to your baby. Before clamping and cutting, you may wish to allow the placenta to pass first.

DELAYED EXAMINATIONS. During the "golden hour"—the first hour after birth—weighing, routine (not required) testing, procedures, and examinations are delayed for about an hour so that mother-baby bonding can begin.

ENVIRONMENT. Providing your baby with a calm, quiet welcome gives you the opportunity to speak to your baby and for them to hear your familiar voice.

EYE TREATMENT. Eye ointment administration is only necessary if you have an active vaginal infection. If this is a state requirement, opt for a *golden hour* delay.

FULL ROOMING-IN. With your baby with you around the clock, you will be better able to notice your baby's hunger cues, which will help you with breastfeeding.

IMMEDIATE SKIN-TO-SKIN CONTACT. Having your baby placed on your chest for immediate skin-to-skin contact has several benefits for mother and newborn, enabling you to breastfeed immediately postpartum.

LOTUS BIRTH. The practice of not cutting the umbilical cord leaves the newborn attached to the placenta until the cord dries naturally and disconnects from the belly button, generally about three days later.

PLACENTA. The placenta will deliver itself without the use of Pitocin or any additional medication. If you like, you can also save the placenta for encapsulation.

VACCINATION. You may choose to delay vaccinations as well. Newborns begin producing vitamin K around the eighth day of life. This medication can be administered orally. The hepatitis B vaccination can also be administered later. If a newborn's mother does not have the virus in her blood, the baby can receive the hepatitis B vaccine *within 24 hours after birth*. When considering whether to vaccinate, set aside a dedicated time to have *several* conversations with your providers *prior* to delivery. If you and your provider agree to an alternate schedule, have the schedule waiver and the details of the alternate schedule placed in your baby's pediatric medical records and keep a copy for yourself.

"Lying-In" Plan

"Lying-In" is a postpartum care practice that lets the mother stay in bed for 40 days after giving birth, while others (specifically family) attend to her needs and those of her household, promoting healing and healthy bonding for the new mom and baby. Sounds great, right? By staying in bed instead of managing household chores and menial tasks, you give your postpartum body the appropriate time and conditions to heal. Lying-in is also a time to strengthen the bond and breastfeeding connection with your newborn. For most women and their families, true lying-in is not realistic, but taking an intentional extended period of rest to focus on healing and connecting with your baby is the ultimate postpartum self-care gift that can be tailored to meet your specific needs.

Delayed Cord Clamping

Delayed umbilical cord clamping (DCC), prolonging the time between the delivery of a newborn and the clamping of the umbilical cord, was originally done only with preterm infants, since they greatly benefitted from the increase in blood volume. However, DCC can actually be beneficial for any infant. The iron in the cord blood increases newborn iron storage, which is vital for optimal brain development in both preterm and full-term babies. Premature infants who receive DCC have better blood pressure in the days immediately after birth and need fewer medical interventions to protect their lives. The benefits of DCC can also be seen later in a child's life, as children whose cords are cut more than three minutes after birth have higher social and fine motor skills than those whose cords were cut within 10 seconds.

Doctors usually follow the World Health Organization's (WHO) recommendation to perform DCC about one minute after delivery; however, most midwives advise women to wait until the cord's pumping stops and the cord turns white. Due to an increase in red blood cells, DCC also decreases the risk of iron-deficiency anemia. Extra blood also helps newborns transition from inside to outside the womb as their lungs receive more blood, making the exchange of oxygen occur smoothly.

Delayed cord clamping is not without some risks. It may result in thick blood and polycythemia, an excess of red blood cells in circulation, which may lead to high levels of bilirubin, a waste product resulting from the breakdown of red blood cells that causes jaundice. Talk to your provider in advance about making the right decision for you and your baby.

Circumcision

As a new parent, you may be very anxious about your baby undergoing this procedure. Male circumcision is a controversial practice involving the surgical removal of the foreskin, or prepuce, that covers the tip of the penis. Attitudes about circumcision are changing amid research and modern ethics, even though it has been the default position for decades in the United States; however, there are a number of medical, religious, and social factors to consider when deciding when and if to circumcise.

Circumcision is a common yet painful procedure and even though complications are rare, there are associated risks. These risks may include prolonged bleeding, infection, and damage to the penis, which may not appear until later in life. These risks are minimal when the procedure is performed by a trained medical professional or mohel in a sterile setting. While some research suggests that circumcision reduces the risk of urinary tract infections, penile- and human papilloma virus (HPV)–related cancers, penile skin conditions, and contracting HIV, maintaining overall good genital hygiene eliminates these risks anyway. Teaching how to keep the penis and genital area clean, with or without foreskin, is imperative. Even though it may not seem obvious to consider how circumcision may affect your baby's sexual sensation as an adult, it is something to keep in mind. Circumcision is permanent, so you owe it to your child to think it through and not leave the decision up to a third party.

If you choose not to circumcise, make sure everyone is aware of your decision. Include this in the birth plan if necessary.

VACCINES

The myth of a causal relationship between pediatric vaccination and autism has disturbingly prompted a number of parents in the United States to opt out of immunizing their children. Twenty-two years ago, Andrew Wakefield, a physician who has since had his medical license revoked, falsely linked the measles, mumps, and rubella (MMR) vaccine to autism in a world-renowned medical journal. The anti-vaccination movement, led by preventive medicine physicians and scientists who embrace this alternative philosophy, is no longer on the fringe. As this faction continues to grow, dispelling myths and correcting misinformation about pediatric immunization is the key to eliminating the risks of contracting and spreading disease.

One of the main anti-vax myths is that vaccines cause autism. Autism is a developmental disorder whose contributing factor is genetics. The Wakefield study that breathed life into this myth was flawed and deemed fraudulent science. It was eventually retracted by its authors because of its intentionally misleading interpretations based on the timing of autism's appearance and the corresponding vaccination schedule. Since then, other, better-designed studies have found no causal link between autism and the MMR vaccine.

Accompanying the causal link myth is the belief that vaccines contain harmful ingredients. Some of the ingredients in vaccinations, like the ingredients in the foods we consume, create an environment for the vaccination to be administered safely, and at doses lower than we are environmentally exposed to every day. Thimerosal, a preservative previously used in multidose vaccination vials, contains ethyl mercury—not *methyl mercury*, which is the form that does damage to the nervous system. As we are naturally exposed to mercury in common products such as milk, seafood, and contact lens solution, the amount of thimerosal used in vaccines poses no more of a health risk than the amount of thimerosal in a can of tuna. Today, routine pediatric vaccines do not contain thimerosal at all.

Some parents erroneously believe that childhood diseases are an integral part of the human life cycle. However, natural infection does not usually cause better immunity than vaccination. Diseases preventable by immunization have serious complications including paralysis, permanent brain damage, organ failure, deafness, blindness, and even death. Immunizations stimulate the immune system to produce a controlled response similar to natural infection, which is not accompanied by potentially devastating complications.

Compulsory vaccination is a concept that has met resistance since the development of the smallpox vaccine in 1796, which cut the death rate from that disease in half in 25 years. Even though immunizations have been proven to be both safe and effective based on high-quality research and scientific evidence, the myths continue to spread. This keeps immunization and anti-vaccination sentiment at the center of controversial debate. Parents and health care professionals alike have biases and misconceptions about the utility of vaccinations. Consequently, it's important to dispel myths and provide substantial evidence that vaccines are safe and necessary.

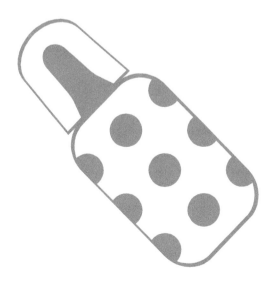

Cloth Diapers

For some mothers, disposable diapers are the go-to option; others champion cloth diapers. Not surprisingly, many environmentally conscious women start off using cloth diapers, but eventually discontinue the practice because, well, it can be time-consuming and exhausting.

Often touted for being a good option for baby's skin, cloth diapers are less absorbent than disposable diapers so they need to be changed more often to avoid diaper rash. Washable diapers are also more cumbersome than their disposable counterparts, which means you may need to buy clothing in a larger size to fit over the extra material. To be a truly green option, cloth diapers need to be washed in full loads, line-dried, and reused on a second child in order to reduce their carbon footprint. For this reason, you will need about twenty cloth diapers if you are planning to use them full-time or mostly full-time. It's a lot. But if it's the right choice for you, it's worth it.

There are several types of cloth diapers and your budget will determine which kind is best for your family. The price of a single cloth diaper ranges from $5 to $20, which means cloth diapers will *eventually* save you money, though the initial investment may be a limiting factor. Cloth diapers are not for everyone; in fact, they may seem like an unlikely alternative for you despite the benefits for the environment. Nevertheless, while cloth diapering is more labor intensive, once you establish a routine, the process gets better as your baby gets older and starts eating solid foods.

Some types of cloth diapers include:

- ALL-IN-ONES, similar to disposable diapers, are one-piece diapering systems that have an inner absorbent layer attached to an outer waterproof layer with adjustable waist closures.

- ALL-IN-TWOS (OR HYBRIDS) are not as bulky as all-in-ones or pocket diapers and are made up of a waterproof outer shell and a detachable insert for absorbency.

- CONTOUR, a two-part diapering system, consists of shapely diapers that fit snugly, have no fasteners, are adjustable at the waist, and need a waterproof diaper cover.

FITTEDS, a highly absorbent option with elastic around the legs to contain leaks. They need a waterproof cover but don't need to be folded.

FLATS are large squares of a single absorbent layer of fabric that need a waterproof diaper cover. They can be folded various ways and fastened with pins.

POCKET, another two-part diapering system, is a diaper cover with an opening for a prefold diaper or insert that can be placed in the opening.

PREFOLDS are rectangular diapers with three panels made from multiple layers of lightweight, gauze-woven fabric with additional layers in the center panel for absorbency.

Breastfeeding

After delivery, your emotions may be unpredictable, especially between days two and five when your milk comes in and the "baby blues" can set in simultaneously. Although nursing might seem like the natural next step after delivery, it doesn't always go smoothly, and it's not always easy. You and your baby will need practice and support during the early weeks. But don't worry! Breastfeeding is a process that can be learned. Though it can be challenging, it's incredibly beneficial to you and your baby.

Exclusively breastfeeding (no formula, juice, or sugar water) for six months will give your baby a healthy start while helping you fend off the symptoms associated with postpartum depression. Two of the best things you can do your first week home is bonding with your baby and getting breastfeeding on track. Breast milk is not only the perfect food for your baby, it also saves money and time. However, breastfeeding can be challenging to keep up, especially if you need to go back to work. You may come to realize that the standard expert recommendations may not be the right fit for you or your baby, either due to personal preferences, lifestyle, and/or poor milk production. If that happens, it's okay. The most important thing is that you do what's right for you and your baby, whatever that turns out to be.

BENEFITS OF BREASTFEEDING

Breastfeeding brings many health benefits to you and your baby, with the reassuring closeness of skin-to-skin contact being the biggest. For as long as you nurse, you and your baby will share a unique bonding opportunity. Breast milk can help protect your baby from allergies and eczema as breast milk proteins are less likely to cause allergic reaction. Breastfeeding also lowers the risk of viral, urinary tract, gastrointestinal, ear, and respiratory infections. The fatty acids in breast milk can also boost neurodevelopment—breastfed babies have higher intelligence quotient scores in early childhood.

Breastfeeding is great for mom, too! As a new mother, watching your baby thrive on your breast milk alone is an empowering experience. Breast-feeding lowers your risk of ovarian and breast cancers and helps you lose pregnancy weight. Milk production not only burns calories, enabling you to avoid dieting, but it also triggers your uterus to return to its pre-pregnancy size. You might even feel contractions while nursing. While breastfeeding, your body absorbs calcium more efficiently, which lowers your risk of post-menopausal osteoporosis. Finally, exclusive breastfeeding prevents ovulation and menstruation, giving you a nonmedicated form of birth control for the first six months of your baby's life.

BABY CUES AND FEEDING PATTERNS

Through breastfeeding, you'll become intimately acquainted with your baby's hunger cues. Even though your baby can't talk, they can let you know when they are ready to eat and when they are full. Although recognizing these subtle cues may take a while, you will learn the signs in no time.

Before crying, your baby will begin to show signs of hunger by moving their hands or fists to their mouth, smacking their lips, and, if you are holding them, searching for your breast. When your baby is full, they will release your breast, turn away from your nipple, relax their body, and/or open their fists. They may also stop nursing without releasing the nipple on their own; if this happens, slide your pinky finger into the corner of their mouth to break the suction seal. Then burp them and offer your other breast. They may nurse again immediately or nurse on the other side later. Frequent nursing also helps you produce enough milk—it's a way to tell your body how much it needs to make for your baby's age and weight.

POSITIONS

Proper breastfeeding positioning is crucial for establishing a physiologically correct latch. For newborns, the LAID-BACK position, with you in a semi-reclining position and your baby lying on your abdomen with their head near your breast, enables your baby to rest on your body in any direction, naturally latching on on their own or with your gentle guidance. The CRADLE HOLD begins with your baby's head positioned in your elbow crease with your hand supporting their body. With your other hand cupping your breast above your nipple (pointing toward your baby's nose), your baby is ready to latch.

The CROSSOVER HOLD starts with you holding your baby's head with the hand opposite the nursing breast. With your free hand, cup your breast for latching. The FOOTBALL HOLD, in contrast, begins with your baby at your side, facing you, with their legs tucked under your arm on the side that you will be nursing. Supporting your baby's head with the same hand, establish the latch in the same way you would for a cradle hold. The SIDE-LYING position, especially useful during night feedings, has you and your baby facing each other, both lying on your sides while cupping your breast as needed.

LATCHING

Getting a good latch is important regardless of which position you use for breastfeeding. Besides helping you feel more comfortable, a good latch will also help your baby efficiently receive milk. To initiate a good latch, tickle your baby's lips with your nipple to stimulate your baby to open their mouth wide. Place your nipple just above your baby's top lip, ensuring that their chin is lifted. Your baby's lips should be flipped outward like a fish, and with their tongue extended, your breast should fill their mouth.

If your baby's initial latch is uncomfortable, gently break the latch with a clean finger and reattempt it. You'll know you have a good latch if you're comfortable and pain-free. You can also check your baby's position, making sure that their chest and stomach are resting against your body, with their head straight and not turned to the side. In addition, you can make sure that your baby's chin touches your breast and their widened mouth encircles your entire breast. If your baby's ears are moving slightly and you can hear (or see) your baby swallowing, you have a good latch.

THE LET-DOWN

When your baby nurses, after about two minutes of suckling, the nerves in your breasts send signals that release the milk from your milk ducts. Called the let-down reflex, this release gets the milk flowing when your baby feeds. You may or may not feel a distinct sensation when it happens, but you should notice a change in your baby's swallowing patterns. During the first few postpartum days before your milk comes in, feeling the let-down reflex may be difficult. In the beginning of breastfeeding, this reflex can be affected by stress, pain, and fatigue, but once regular feeding is established, you're off to the races.

If you are having trouble with let-down, first try to relax with the breathing techniques you used during labor. Eliminate distractions and disruptions by going to a place where you can be alone to focus solely on your baby. In some potentially embarrassing cases, mothers with sensitive let-down reflexes will hear a crying baby or merely think of their baby and will experience a let-down reflex even if they are not nursing. Gentle breast massages, warm compresses on your breasts, and warm showers will also help initiate the let-down reflex if you are having continued challenges.

PUMPING AND BOTTLES

You may choose not to breastfeed for physical, social, or personal reasons, even if you believe that breast milk is the best food for your child. Pumping is a great way to provide your baby with your breast milk without physically nursing. Whereas all breast pumps extract milk from your breasts, some do so automatically (electric, battery-operated, and hands-free) and others are like hand pumps that work manually.

Although you don't have to sterilize your pump after every session, you should sterilize it before using it for the first time. You may also want to sanitize your pump if your baby is under three months old or if they are immunocompromised. To clean and sterilize your pump parts, just run it in the dishwasher with hot water and the heated drying cycle.

To store your pumped milk, use breast milk storage bags or glass storage containers with tight-fitting lids. You can use plastic storage containers for storage if you avoid BPA-containing plastic bottles with the recycle symbol number 7. Freshly pumped milk can be stored at room temperature for up to four hours, in the refrigerator for up to four days, and in the freezer for up to one year.

DIET AND NUTRITION

A general rule is that you can eat anything in moderation while breast-feeding; however, calorie restriction and other weight loss methods will negatively affect your milk supply. Barley increases prolactin, the breast-feeding hormone, and can be used in soups, stews, and salads. Fennel and fenugreek contain phytoestrogens that help milk production, though women with diabetes, heart disease, or nut allergies should consult their doctor before adding fenugreek to their diets. Raw fennel, tossed with olive oil and balsamic vinegar, pairs well with grapefruit, orange, and mint, while cooked fennel pairs well with roasted chicken and fish.

After barley, oats are the most well-known breast milk booster. They can be crumbled on top of fruit or muffins and baked in cookies. Whole wheat and brown rice are also great, and easily overlooked because they are dietary staples. Brewer's yeast, a breast milk booster often found in lactation cook-ies, passes readily into breast milk. Unfortunately, the bitter taste may cause gastrointestinal discomfort in infants. Papaya, raw and cooked in soups, can be used with yogurt, cereal, fruit salad, and noodle dishes to help increase supply. Breastfeeding women should limit their intake of caffeine, alcohol, and cow's milk, as these foods decrease milk supply.

BREASTFEEDING AND POSTPARTUM DEPRESSION (PPD)

In our reproductive medicine and women's health practice, we encourage mothers to breastfeed exclusively. Breastfeeding is not only the most affordable option for families, it also encourages bonding in a unique way that benefits both the mother and the baby. In general, breastfeeding tends to be more successful among mothers with more support and fewer life stressors. Many new mothers come to our practice for help with breastfeeding challenges. Unlike most practices, which mainly examine the infant's mouth and the mother's breasts looking for structural problems that could affect breastfeeding, we explore the psychological effects of not being able to breastfeed. We also make an internal referral to our lactation consultant.

For many mothers, breastfeeding is one of the things they look forward to the most. We also see women who do not want to breastfeed and move through motherhood just fine. We see women who become emotionally distraught because they were committed to breastfeeding but ran into challenges, like unplanned cesareans, delivery complications, infants with medical issues, and difficulties with breastfeeding itself.

Our practitioners recognize the extreme pressure that women place on themselves to breastfeed. Some may become discouraged and depressed. However, sometimes *you,* the patient, may not even realize that you are experiencing symptoms of depression. Even though some mothers experience positive feelings when breastfeeding, you may not. If you are too tired to make decisions about your hygiene or your infant's, this could be indicative of PPD. Your health care team can work with you to address PPD in a timely manner while helping you reach your breastfeeding goals. They can also help you find treatment options for depression, including medications and nonpharmacological options like acupuncture, herbal therapy, and individual or group therapy, along with professional breastfeeding support as needed. When breastfeeding becomes more challenging than anticipated—like when you're struggling with latching on or with a painful latch—your milk supply is compromised, which often leads to supplementing with formula. For a mom committed to breastfeeding, this can lead to feelings of shame, guilt, inadequacy as a mother, and depression.

In general, mothers want the best for their babies, so difficulty breastfeeding may lead to significant amounts of stress. This stress may manifest in feelings of sadness, hopelessness, and worry; however, when these feelings last longer than two weeks, this may be more than just a dip in mood. If feelings of sadness and guilt lead to frequent crying spells, this could be a red flag, especially if coupled with a loss of interest in the activities that you typically enjoy, as well as drastically altered sleep patterns. Thoughts of harming yourself or your baby are an advanced sign of PPD and possibly postpartum psychosis. If you have these kinds of thoughts, talk to your provider immediately and contact Postpartum Support International at 800-944-4PPD (4773) to get the help you need. If you experience symptoms associated with PPD, you can still achieve your breastfeeding goals with an adequate support system, socially and clinically.

Swaddling

Finding the best swaddle for your baby can be a lifesaver. A good swaddle can help your baby feel secure, as they did in the comfort, safety, warmth, and snugness of the womb. When done correctly and safely, with babies who do not co-sleep and are not turning over yet, swaddling benefits you and your baby. Swaddled babies sleep longer and sleep more soundly. They also experience less anxiety. Swaddling prevents your infant from unnecessary wake-ups due to the startle reflex. It also eliminates the need for comfort items in your baby's crib that have been linked to sudden infant death syndrome (SIDS).

Ultimately, swaddling in the hands-over-heart position is the preferred sleeping position for your infant. In this position, babies learn to self-soothe and return to sleep on their own. Wearing a swaddle helps maintain baby's back-sleeping position while reminding you to place your baby on their back when sleeping.

DIAMOND SWADDLE

On a safe, flat surface, position the blanket in a diamond, fold down the top corner, and place your baby on the blanket with their head above the fold. With their right arm by their side, wrap the right corner of the blanket across their chest, tucking it behind their back on the left. Place their left arm by their side and wrap the left corner of the blanket across their chest, securing it under their back on the right. Take the bottom corner of the blanket up and over their body and tuck it under their chin, ensuring that no fabric covers their mouth or nose.

SQUARE SWADDLE

Lay a blanket down in a square shape. Fold the top right corner down about four to six inches. This is where you will place your baby's head. Lay your baby down on the blanket on their back with their neck at the top of the fold. They will be lying diagonally across the blanket. Pull the right side over and snugly tuck it under their body, making sure they are in the frog leg position (legs bent and turned out) and their hips are loose. Pull the left side over their body and snugly tuck it under them. Lastly, tuck the bottom of the blanket behind them.

SLEEP SACK SWADDLE

For babies who resist the conventional swaddle, you may want to opt for a sleep sack swaddle. To safely use a sleep sack swaddle, dress your baby in their regular sleepwear and close the zipper. Fold the left swaddle wing over your baby's torso and right arm, then tuck the tip of the wing under your baby's left arm. Fold the right swaddle wing over your baby's torso and left arm, fastening the Velcro over your baby's right arm. Make sure the swaddle wrap is snug, below the chin, and parallel to your baby's shoulders.

Co-sleeping

With so many stark opinions on both sides of the discussion, *co-sleeping* and *bed-sharing* have become hot topics. Although co-sleeping and bed-sharing are often used interchangeably, they do not have the same meaning. Bed-sharing means that you share the same sleeping surface with your baby. Co-sleeping means that your baby sleeps in close proximity to you, on the same surface or not. Using this definition, co-sleeping is actually a form of *room-sharing*. Room-sharing, recommended until your baby is at least six months old, minimizes the risk of sudden infant death syndrome (SIDS). For this reason, in our practice we prefer not to use the term "co-sleeping," instead using "bed-sharing" and "room-sharing," which have clear definitions.

Keeping your baby within view is the most important thing to remember when sharing your room with your baby. Baby boxes, which are just portable cardboard bassinets, are often baby's first sleeping space and can be used for about five months. They are safe places where your newborn can immediately sleep upon their arrival to your home, which simultaneously reduces the need for bed-sharing and the risk of SIDS. Put your baby's crib or bassinet wherever you can clearly see them and reach them quickly to feed and soothe your baby when necessary. White noise, in the form of a fan, drowns out other noises and can serve as a sleep signal. The use of a fan can also lower the risk of SIDS.

Lactation-Friendly Postpartum Recipes

OATMEAL LACTATION COOKIES

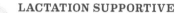

LACTATION SUPPORTIVE

MAKES 24 COOKIES / PREP TIME: 20 MINUTES / COOK TIME: 15 MINUTES

Hooray for a cookie that's good for you! This recipe is packed with nutritious ingredients, including three key ingredients that can help support lactation: flaxseed, brewer's yeast, and oats. These cookies are also free of wheat, dairy, and white sugar for those who may have sensitivities to these foods. They also freeze well. This is a perfect recipe to make in bulk ahead of your delivery date.

2 tablespoons ground flaxseed

6 tablespoons water

3 tablespoons brewer's yeast

1 cup almond flour

½ cup tapioca flour

1 teaspoon baking powder

½ teaspoon sea salt

¾ cup coconut sugar (if you can't find this, use brown sugar instead)

1 teaspoon cinnamon

1 large egg

¼ cup coconut oil, melted

1 teaspoon vanilla extract

1. Preheat the oven to 350°F.
2. Mix the ground flaxseed with the water and let sit for at least 10 minutes.
3. In a bowl, mix together the brewer's yeast, almond flour, tapioca flour, baking powder, salt, coconut sugar, and cinnamon.
4. In a separate bowl, whisk the egg and add it to the dry ingredients.
5. Add in the flaxseed-water mixture.
6. Add in the melted coconut oil and the vanilla extract. Mix well.
7. Add in the oats, and the chocolate chips and raisins (if using). Stir to combine.

2½ cups rolled oats

Mix-in options: ¾ cup chocolate chips and 1 cup raisins. You can also try dried cranberries, walnuts, or chopped pecans. Choose two of your favorites.

8. Scoop out large spoonfuls of the dough and place them on a cookie tray lined with parchment paper (or greased with coconut oil), at least 1 inch apart from one another.

9. Bake for 12 minutes. Let cool before serving.

PER SERVING (1 cookie): Calories: 125; Total fat: 6g; Saturated fat: 2g; Cholesterol: 7mg; Sodium: 88mg; Carbohydrates: 16g; Fiber: 2g; Protein: 4g

MAKE-AHEAD TIP: These are even great frozen. Make a few batches ahead of time and freeze to have on hand for a quick, nutritious snack. If you make them in bulk, the mix-in options add some variety that's tailored to your postpartum tastes.

CHOCOLATE-ALMOND BUTTER SMOOTHIE

LACTATION SUPPORTIVE, QUICK AND EASY

SERVES 2 / PREP TIME: 5 MINUTES

Smoothies are an excellent way to pack in enough calories (and good quality ones) when you are breastfeeding. This recipe satisfies the taste buds, provides healthy fats and fiber, and even includes a few ingredients, like fennel seed and brewer's yeast, to help with breast milk production.

1 cup unsweetened almond milk

1 tablespoon almond butter

½ teaspoon fennel seeds

½ teaspoon brewer's yeast

¼ avocado

1 teaspoon vanilla extract

1 tablespoon cocoa powder

1 medium banana

2 dates

1 cup ice

Put the almond milk, almond butter, fennel seed, brewer's yeast, avocado, vanilla extract, cocoa powder, banana, dates, and ice into a blender. Blend well and serve immediately.

PER SERVING: Calories: 186; Total fat: 9g; Saturated fat: 1g; Cholesterol: 0mg; Sodium: 92mg; Carbohydrates: 25g; Fiber: 6g; Protein: 5g

SUBSTITUTION TIP: You can swap the almond butter for peanut butter or sunflower butter. If you would like this smoothie sweeter, add more dates.

CREAMY BLACK BEAN SOUP

LACTATION SUPPORTIVE, PROTEIN POWER, VEGGIE LOADED

SERVES 8 / PREP TIME: 30 MINUTES / COOK TIME: 45 MINUTES

This creamy black bean soup provides nourishment to help support you in the postpartum phase. It has vegetables, healthy fats, and protein. The fennel seeds add a nice flavor, are soothing to the digestive system, and help support breast milk production.

1 tablespoon extra-virgin olive oil

½ medium onion, chopped

3 garlic cloves, minced

2 medium celery stalks, chopped

1 carrot, chopped

1 teaspoon sea salt

2 teaspoons fennel seeds

2 (15-ounce) cans black beans, drained and rinsed

2 (32-ounce) containers chicken or vegetable broth

1 cup canned coconut milk

1 avocado, sliced

1. In a soup pot, heat the olive oil over medium-high heat.
2. Add the onion and cook for about 2 minutes.
3. Add the garlic, celery, carrot, salt, and fennel seeds and sauté for 5 minutes or until cooked through.
4. Add the beans and broth and bring to a boil. Cover and let simmer for 30 minutes so the flavors can blend.
5. Put half the soup into a blender. Add the coconut milk and blend.
6. Place the blended mixture back into the soup pot and stir to combine.
7. Serve with sliced avocado.

PER SERVING: Calories: 228; Total fat: 11g; Saturated fat: 5g; Cholesterol: 5mg; Sodium: 1,299mg; Carbohydrates: 27g; Fiber: 10g; Protein: 8g

PREP TIP: You can use dried black beans instead of canned and cook them in a digital pressure cooker: 1) cover 1½ cups of dried black beans with water and soak overnight, 2) drain the beans and transfer to a digital pressure cooker, 3) cover the beans with water by 2 inches, 4) use the bean/legume setting, which should be about 20 minutes of pressure cooking, and 5) for step 4 above, add in the cooked beans and their broth instead of the chicken/vegetable broth. The freshly cooked beans add a wonderful flavor to this soup.

Essential Oil Blends
for Breastfeeding

In this section you'll find some essential oil blends that can assist with breastfeeding and other common postpartum issues.

BREASTFEEDING

Clary Sage, Basil, and Geranium essential oils can help stimulate breast milk production. Fennel essential oil works to increase your breast milk supply. Using Fennel oil for long periods of time can negatively affect the urinary tract, however, so you should limit use to less than 10 days. To prepare these essential oils, blend 5 to 10 drops with a tablespoon of coconut oil and then apply the blend to your breast or lymph area to boost your milk supply. Do not apply oil directly to your nipple just before nursing, as your baby may be repulsed by the scent and taste.

SORE NIPPLES

Sore, cracked, or dry nipples can occur when breastfeeding. Even though breast milk heals sore nipples, you can use Frankincense, Lavender, Geranium, Roman Chamomile, and Neroli essential oils for additional help with healing and discomfort. Immediately after nursing, rub 6 to 10 drops of one of these oils on your affected nipples after mixing with one tablespoon of coconut or almond oil. Massage the oil blend on the sore nipples and areola. Be sure to rinse your nipples before the next feeding so your baby does not ingest any of the oil. Myrrh, Sandalwood, and Wild Orange essential oils can also help.

INSOMNIA

To soothe, calm, and combat insomnia, mix 15 drops of Lavender essential oil, 10 drops of Vetiver essential oil, and 5 drops each of Frankincense, Orange, and Ylang Ylang essential oils together and dilute with five tablespoons of coconut carrier oil. As an alternative to topical, you can also use essential oil blends in a bath. Mix one drop each of Lavender essential oil and Sweet Marjoram essential oil with two drops of Roman Chamomile essential oil. When using essential oils in a bath, use no more than six to eight drops total, according to your aromatic preferences.

ANXIETY

Taking a relaxing bath in the morning or in the evening can relieve anxiety symptoms. Mix two drops of Clary Sage essential oil, three drops each of Lavender and Ylang Ylang essential oils, and two drops each of Roman Chamomile and Marjoram essential oils in two tablespoons of your preferred carrier oil and add to your bath. As an inhalation, hold an open bottle of 5 drops each of Bergamot and Neroli essential oils and 10 drops of Lavender oil with an ounce of carrier oil a few inches away from your noise and waft the scent toward your nose.

Conclusion

Thank you for the invitation to join you on your pregnancy and childbirth journey! You are well on your way to creating a happy home. Parenting will be stressful at times as motherhood now welcomes you with the new challenge of work-life balance. Balancing the demands of motherhood, family, friendships, and career may often feel like an impossible feat, but keep it in perspective—despite the challenges, you have already successfully completed one of the hardest jobs a woman can complete: you gave birth.

As you continue life as a parent, know that you will continue to make healthy choices for you, your child, and your family. Be confident in yourself as you embrace your new role. As the central pillar of your family, make the commitment to keep yourself healthy mentally, physically, and spiritually. Continue eating wisely, exercising, surrounding yourself with supportive people, and engaging in nurturing activities that build you up. Trust your instincts. Even when you do not know exactly what to do, lead with love, and you will find yourself on the correct path. Tend to your own needs by taking care of yourself so that you will be able to fully enjoy the joys of your baby and the new family that you created. Remember to live in the present, enjoying all the precious moments you are experiencing. Wishing you continued health, wellness, and flourishing as you embark on the next phase of your journey.

Until we meet again . . . Salud!

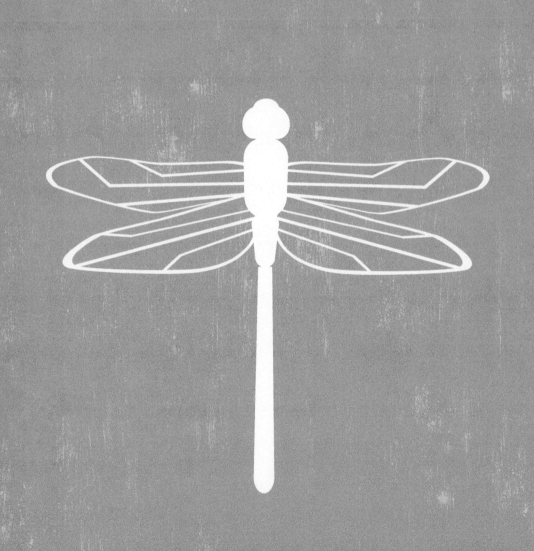

References

American College of Obstetricians and Gynecologists. *Your Pregnancy and Birth*. 4th ed. Washington, DC: Meredith Books, 2005.

Bradley, Christine F. "Psychological Consequences of Intervention in the Birth Process." *Canadian Journal of Behavioural Science / Revue canadienne des sciences du comportement* 15, no. 4 (1983): 422–38, doi.org/10.1037/h0080762.

Campbell, Della, Marian Lake, Michele Falk, and Jeffrey Backstrand. "A Randomized Control Trial of Continuous Support in Labor by a Lay Doula." *Journal of Obstetric, Gynecologic and Neonatal Nursing* 35, no. 4 (Jul.–Aug. 2006): 456–64, doi: 10.1111/j.1552-6909.2006.00067.x.

Ceriani Cernadas, José M., Guillermo Carroli, Liliana Pellegrini, Lucas Otaño, Marina Ferreira, Carolina Ricci, Ofelia Casas, et al. "The Effect of Timing of Cord Clamping on Neonatal Venous Hematocrit Values and Clinical Outcome at Term: A Randomized, Controlled Trial." *Pediatrics* 117, no. 4 (2006): e779-e786. doi:10.1542/peds.2005-1156.

Curtis, Glade B, and Judith Schuler. *Your Pregnancy Week by Week*. 4th ed. Cambridge, MA: Da Capo Lifelong Books, 2000.

Devereaux, Yolanda, and Henline Sullivan. "Doula Support While Laboring: Does it Help Achieve a More Natural Birth?" *International Journal of Childbirth Education* 28, no. 2 (Apr. 2013): 54–61.

Ellison, Michael. *10 Habits of Wellness For a Happier and Healthier Life with Less Illness*. Scottsdale, AZ: TriVita Press, 2019.

Emerson, William R. "Birth Trauma: The Psychological Effects of Obstetrical Interventions." *Journal of Prenatal & Perinatal Psychology & Health* 13, no. 1 (1998): 11–44.

Environmental Working Group. "EWG's 10 Tips for a Less Toxic Pregnancy." Last modified December 7, 2009. Ewg.org/enviroblog/2009/12/ewgs-10-tips-less-toxic-pregnancy.

Garabedian, Charles, Thameur Rakza, Elodie Drumez, Marion Poleszczuk, Louise Ghesquiere, Bénédicte Wibaut, M. H. Depoortere, et al. "Benefits of Delayed Cord Clamping in Red Blood Cell Alloimmunization." *Pediatrics* 137, no. 3 (Mar. 2016): e20153236, doi:10.1542/peds.2015-3236.

Green, Jeanne, and Barbara A. Hotelling. "Healthy Birth Practice #3: Bring a Loved One, Friend, or Doula for Continuous Support." *Journal of Perinatal Education* 28, no. 2 (Apr. 2019), doi:10.1891/1058-1243.28.2.88.

Hodnett, Ellen D., and Richard W. Osborn. "Effects of Continuous Intrapartum Professional Support on Childbirth Outcomes." *Research in Nursing & Health* 12, no. 5 (Oct. 1989): 289–97, doi:10.1002/nur.4770120504.

Hviid, Anders, Jørgen Vinsløv Hansen, Morten Frisch, and Mads Melbye. "Measles, Mumps, Rubella Vaccination and Autism: A Nationwide Cohort Study." *Annals of Internal Medicine* 170 (Apr. 2019): 513–20, doi:10.7326/M18-2101.

Kavosi, Zahra, Ali Keshtkaran, Fatemeh Setoodehzadeh, Maryam Kasraeian, Mohammad Khammarnia, and Marzieh Eslahi. "A Comparison of Mothers' Quality of Life after Normal Vaginal, Cesarean, and Water Birth Deliveries." *International Journal of Community Based Nursing and Midwifery* 3, no. 3 (Jul. 2015): 198–204.

Kemp, Melissa L., and Beth Hart. "MMR Vaccine and Autism: Is There a Link?" *Journal of the American Academy of PAs* 23, no. 6 (Jun. 2010): 48–50.

Kennell, John, Marshall Klaus, and Susan McGrath. "Continuous Emotional Support during Labor in a US Hospital: A Randomized Controlled Trial." *Journal of the American Medical Association* 265, no. 17 2197–201, doi:10.1001/jama.1991.03460170051032.

Kozhimannil, Katy B., Laura B. Attanasio, Judy Jou, Lauren K. Joarnt, Pamela J. Johnson, and Dwenda K. Gjerdingen. "Potential Benefits of Increased Access to Doula Support during Childbirth." *American Journal of Managed Care* 20, no. 8 (Aug. 2014): e340–e352.

Lee, Kathryn A., and Caryl L. Gay. "Sleep in Late Pregnancy Predicts Length of Labor and Type of Delivery." *American Journal of Obstetrics & Gynecology* 191, no. 6 (2004): 2041-6, doi: 10.1016/j.ajog.2004.05.086.

Lipson, Julienne G., and Virginia P. Tilden. "Psychological Integration of the Cesarean Birth Experience. *American Journal of Orthopsychiatry* 50, no. 4 (1980): 598–609, doi: 10.1111/j.1939-0025.1980.tb03322.x.

McAdams, Ryan M. "Time to Implement Delayed Cord Clamping." *Obstetrics & Gynecology* 123, no. 3 (Mar. 2014): 549–52, doi:10.1097/AOG.0000000000000122.

Murkoff, Heidi, and Sharon Mazel. *What to Expect When You're Expecting.* 4th ed. New York: Workman Publishing Company, 2008.

Noyman-Veksler, Gal, Shirley Herishanu-Gilutz, Ora Kofman, Gershon Holchberg, and Golan Shahar. "Post-natal Psychopathology and Bonding with the Infant among First-Time Mothers Undergoing a Caesarian Section and Vaginal Delivery: Sense of Coherence and Social Support as Moderators." *Psychology and Health* 30, no. 4 (Apr. 2015): 441–55, doi:10.1080 /08870446.2014.977281.

Olza, Ibone, Patricia Leahy-Warren, Yael Benyamini, Maria Kazmierczak, Sigfridur Ina Karlsdottir, Andria Spyridou, Esther Crespo-Mirasol, et al. "Women's Psychological Experiences of Physiological Childbirth: A Meta-synthesis." *BMJ Open* 8 (2018): e020347, doi:10.1136/bmjopen -2017-020347.

Raju, Tonse N. K. "Timing of Umbilical Cord Clamping after Birth for Optimizing Placental Transfusion." *Current Opinion in Pediatrics* 25, no. 2 (Apr. 2013): 180–87, doi: 10.1097/MOP.0b013e32835d2a9e.

Simkin, Penny. "Pain, Suffering, and Trauma in Labor and Prevention of Subsequent Posttraumatic Stress Disorder." *The Journal of Perinatal Education* 20, no. 3 (Summer 2011): 166–76, doi:10.1891/1058-1243.20.3.166.

Stein, Martin T. "Benefits of a Doula Present at the Birth of a Child." *Pediatrics* 114, no. 6 (2004): 1488–91, doi:10.1542/peds.2004-1721R.

Steingraber, Sandra. *Having Faith: An Ecologist's Journey to Motherhood.* New York: The Berkeley Publishing Group, 2003.

Thurston, Lydia A. Futch, Dalia Abrams, Alexa Dreher, Stephanie R. Ostrowski, and James C. Wright. "Improving Birth and Breastfeeding Outcomes among Low Resource Women in Alabama by Including Doulas in the Interprofessional Birth Care Team." *Journal of Interprofessional Education & Practice* 17 (Dec. 2019), doi: 10.1016/j.xjep.2019.100278.

Verdult, Rien. "Cesarean Birth: Psychological Aspects in Adults." *International Journal of Prenatal and Perinatal Psychology and Medicine* 21, no. 1/2 (2009): 17–36.

Index

Acknowledgments

Five years ago, even as people suggested that I write a book, I scoffed at the notion. Now, at the completion of my debut book, I am so happy that I accepted the challenge, as it has been more rewarding than I could have ever imagined. None of this would have been possible without the love and support of . . . my people.

Always, forever, and foremost, thank you to Jesus Christ, my Lord and Savior, who has blessed me with the gifts that have allowed me to follow my calling, persevere, and fulfill my purpose in life.

I am eternally grateful for my parents, Joan and Laurence White Sr., who have sustained me and NEVER cease to love me, support me, and BELIEVE IN ME and my *wild* dreams even when they do not truly understand me (or them). They each have taught me so much that has helped me succeed in life. I truly have no idea where I would be without them. They have stood by me during every struggle (and there have been many) and all my successes. Love you both!

For my aunt and godmother, Lucille Woods, who constantly motivates me with her patience, kindness, work ethic, and compassion. Your intellect inspires me to keep my own mind sharp. Thank you for continuing to be a positive influence and a role model. Love you!

To my youngest brother and biggest fan, Jordan White. You have always cheered me on, encouraged me, and never let me quit. I love you and thank you!

For my nephew, Braxton Lassiter, for holding me accountable to my words and deeds. You, nephew, inspire me to be and do better each day. Love you!

To my girl, Dr. Tiffany Lovelace, for always telling me how proud she is, and encouraging me to stay focused and push all the distractions to the left.

For Jan Bull, who is probably freaking out right now because she made the cut on these acknowledgments. I am so grateful for our friendship because watching you evolve has reminded me of your *promise*. Continue to be a loving light.

To my superstar friend, Keli Garza, who inspires me and encourages me to be better each day through her passion, work, and service.

A heartfelt thank you to my sisterhood at The Eudaimonia Center who decided to join me on this adventure of revolutionizing women's health and "nourishing the flourish" in me, one another, and our patients/clients. Thank you for allowing my powerful, radiant, life-giving joy to shine. To:

April Cohen, for being a continual spiritual guide and compass

Allegra Estreet, for reminding me of my simultaneous "superwoman-ness" and "human-ness"

Yvette Gause, for lovingly welcoming me into her family

Jocelyn Johnson, for inspiring me with her courage and bravery

Anna Schoonover, for being an invaluable resource to our team

Kai Potts Smith, for being a fellow Taurus who just "gets me"

Gabriela Van Sickle, for challenging me intellectually and strengthening my professional skills as a practitioner

Charissa Zhu, for accepting my most challenging requests with ease and completing them efficiently

For countless teachers and mentors, I appreciate the time and effort you took to teach me and help me during the learning process.

Finally, to all our patients and clients, THANK YOU for believing in our genuinely integrative approach to reproductive medicine and women's health, wellness, and healing. Because of you, I have renewed energy as I wake up each morning to go to work. I not only love WHAT I do, I love HOW I am able to do it. You are a source of inspiration and encouragement. Thank you for inviting me to join you on your healing journeys.

About the Author

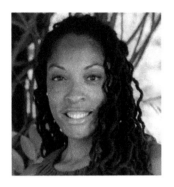

DR. LAURENA WHITE has more than 20 years of service and experience in the field of women's health, ranging from birth doula to obstetrics/gynecology and reproductive endocrinology/infertility to acupuncture and Chinese herbal medicine. She works closely with a carefully designed team to deliver expert care to women experiencing complex health challenges such as uterine fibroids, polycystic ovarian syndrome, endometriosis, hormone imbalances, chronic fatigue syndrome, menopause, menstrual dysfunction, and fibromyalgia. She and her team treat not only women but also couples who are experiencing fertility challenges and are trying to conceive. Dr. White and her team facilitate the transformation of complex women's health and fertility challenges by helping women and couples address the underlying root cause of their respective conditions. Using purpose-built signature programs that are unique to The Eudaimonia Center, her patients and clientele begin to flourish without taking unnecessary pharmaceutical medications and synthetic hormones or having fruitlessly invasive surgical procedures.

Dr. White integrated her practice by forming a synergistic marriage between allopathic and traditional Chinese medicine treatment modalities in order to bridge the gaps in women's health care.

In her personal time, Dr. White enjoys practicing capoeira, cooking, reading, traveling, and basking in the warm rays of the sun at the beach with her family and friends.

CPSIA information can be obtained
at www.ICGtesting.com
Printed in the USA
BVHW091438141020
590860BV00001B/1

9 781647 397074